Legal Aspects
Management

Note

Healthcare practice and knowledge are constantly changing and developing as new research and treatments, changes in procedures, drugs and equipment become available.

The author and publishers have, as far as is possible, taken care to confirm that the information complies with the latest standards of practice and legislation.

Legal Aspects of Pain Management

Second edition

British Journal of Nursing monograph
Legal Aspects of Health Care series

Bridgit Dimond

MA, LLB, DSA, AHSM, Barrister-at-law,
Emeritus Professor of the University of Glamorgan

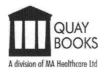

QUAY
BOOKS
A division of MA Healthcare Ltd

Quay Books Division, MA Healthcare Ltd, St Jude's Church, Dulwich Road, London
SE24 0PB

British Library Cataloguing-in-Publication Data
A catalogue record is available for this book

© MA Healthcare Limited 2010

ISBN-10: 1-85642-395-6
ISBN-13: 978-1-85642-395-3

Printed by CLE, Huntingdon, Cambridgeshire

Contents

Foreword

Ilora G. Finlay Finlay, FRCP FRCGP

Pain is perhaps the most feared of all the sensations. It generates fear and despair, breaks the victim in its wake and tortures the onlooker, be that family or friend. Old fears of morphine as a potent and potentially lethal drug gave way in the 1970s to a realisation that the drug was an effective analgesic. When administered orally and titrated up to achieve analgesia, it provides pain relief without shortening life. Yet the abuses became evident in society with addiction, tales of 'double effect' and the murderous intent of Shipman.

Lessons from other countries are important. The legalisation of euthanasia in Holland, until recently not legalised but simply not prosecuted when administered within guidelines, has resulted in a swing back amongst professionals. Awareness of the need for palliative care education and training has increased and doctors are realising that every single patient needs to be able to access good symptom control. As Robert Twycross so often said, 'You do not need to kill the patient to kill the pain.'

The law can seem a blunt instrument when a clinician confronts the myriad of clinical issues in any one patient and tries, sometimes without success, to come to a sound decision in the patient's best interest. We can all learn from the precedents that have made case law. European law is now supplementing this legal framework in England and Wales; it is increasingly shaping the attitudes of society to clinical decision-making processes. Yet lawyers often seem terrifying to clinicians, as if they are ready to pounce on any error to make capital out of it, ignorant of the difficulties and uncertainties the clinician faces, as the law appears to set absolutes that may be open to misinterpretation. Patient autonomy is a phrase much bandied about. Often forgotten is the irrefutable principle that each person is autonomous and the autonomy of one cannot override the autonomy of another within the principles of bio-medical ethics.

The contextual legal framework, within which care is delivered to those who are suffering, highlights why failure to respect the duty of care has severe consequences in law. This book sensitively takes the clinical scenario and explores it, providing references and teaching challenges for discussion. For the next generation of healthcare professionals decisions will become harder, not easier. The internet with its information explosion creates new challenges as patients and their families can access vast mounts of unclassified information; some is based on sound scientific enquiry, some is based on validated human experience. But amongst the 'information' of 'pseudo- information' is much that is simply whim or exploitation of the vulnerable. It is through this minefield that the clinician must steer the person in distress. And as increasingly difficult decisions are taken, ignorance of the law is no defence.

Preface

I welcomed the opportunity to bring this small book up to date. Much has happened in both statute and common law since the First Edition. In particular the Mental Capacity Act 2005 has at long last filled the gap which existed in statute law on decision making on behalf of those incapable of making their own decisions. The aims of the book remain the same: to bring an understanding of the law relating to the management of pain to the many health and social care professionals, including their managers and their tutors in an easy to read succinct way. I also hope that the book will be useful to patients and patient representatives and their organisations. If practitioners have confidence in the law which applies to their practice, then they can concentrate on their work of caring for the patient. If patients understand the law which applies to their situation and their legal rights, then their dialogue with their health and social care professionals can be constructive and meaningful.

Bridgit Dimond

Preface to the First Edition

In 1987 I was seconded from the then Polytechnic of Wales (now the University of Glamorgan) to work with South Glamorgan Health Authority and during that time acted as patient's representative at the Cardiff Royal Infirmary. During my work there we set up several multidisciplinary brainstorming groups to resolve intractable problems in the hospital. One of these was the difficulties of patients who had come to the Accident and Emergency Department with injuries or conditions which required the examination by doctors from other specialities in the hospital, such as paediatrics, orthopaedics, etc. It was the policy that pain relief should not be administered by the Accident and Emergency staff until the patient had been seen by the specialist doctor. Unfortunately this could involve seriously long waiting times for the patients and the situation was clearly unacceptable. One of the members of the brainstorming group was Ann Taylor, a nurse from the Intensive Care Unit. Subsequently, she developed an interest in pain management and moved from the Cardiff Royal Infirmary to the University Hospital of Wales, where she now works in the Department of Anaesthetics and Intensive Care. She initiated an international course for multidisciplinary health professionals in pain management and this has since been developed to Masters degree status with other lecturers involved. Ann's work in this field was subsequently recognised when she was appointed as Welsh Woman of the Year in 1999.

It has been my privilege to give the legal input to the course and it has always been evident to me that a book covering the legal aspects of pain management would be a useful adjunct not only to those on the pain management course and other similar courses, but to all those many health professional from a wide range of specialities who have to deal with many complex legal issues relating to pain management. It should also be of benefit to patient groups and relatives and others involved in palliative care. This book is written for all such people. Because of the variety of their disciplines, the generic term (pain) practitioner will be used, and because the majority are female 'she' and 'her' will be used to denote an individual. Many readers may not be acquainted with basic facts of the legal system and so these are briefly set out in early chapters. It is hoped that the book will provide a succinct, useful basis from which practitioners and others can extend their knowledge of the law for the protection of their patients, their colleagues and themselves. In recognition of the origins of these writings and her significant work in pain management, the book is dedicated to Ann Taylor.

Bridgit Dimond

Acknowledgements

Many people have assisted me in the preparation of this book, particularly those who have participated in the Diploma and Masters Courses in Pain Management run by the Welsh National School of Medicine, with their many questions and concerns about legal issues.

In addition, I am considerably indebted to the help of Ann Taylor and her colleagues, to Elizabeth Holden, Carys Evans and Joanne Larkman with their assistance on benefits available to those receiving palliative care, and to Pat Simpson for her many ideas. As always I am grateful to the constant support and encouragement of Bette Griffiths who once again prepared the indexes.

To Ann

CHAPTER I

The legal system

Box 1.1: Situation

June was suffering from multiple sclerosis (MS) and experiencing considerable pain. She learnt from an MS support group that fellow sufferers had successfully used cannabis to control the pain. She was given information about how she could obtain it, but was warned that it was contrary to the law and that she could face imprisonment. She decided to take the risk. Unfortunately, she was caught while making the purchase and she and the drug dealer were arrested. June feels that there should not be a law making it illegal for her to have pain relief and is worried about whether she could be sent to gaol. What is the situation?

What is 'law'?

How was any law created to make an MS sufferer taking cannabis a criminal?

Our laws derive from two principal sources: Acts of Parliament/Statutory Instruments (known as statute or legislation) and decided cases. (See Glossary for further explanations of legal terms). For further information on all aspects of law covered in the book readers are referred to the author's book (Dimond, 2008) and the other works cited in the further reading section on p. 177.

Legislation

Legislation, as well as consisting of Acts of Parliament (approval by the Houses of Commons and Lords and the Queen's signature) would also include directives and regulations emanating from the European Community, which the UK, as a member state, is required to implement and obey (see below).

Legislation can be primary or secondary. Primary legislation consists of Acts of Parliament, known as Statutes, which come into force at a date set either in the initial Act of Parliament or a date subsequently fixed by order of a Minister (i.e. by Statutory Instrument). The date of enforcement is often later than the date it is passed by the two Houses of Parliament and signed by the Crown. The statute sometimes gives power to a Minister to enact more detailed laws and this is known as secondary legislation. Statutory Instruments that are quoted in the text are an example of this secondary legislation. Referring to the situation in *Box 1.1*, it is as a result of legislation, in particular the Misuse of Drugs Act 1971, that the use of cannabis is at the time of writing a criminal offence. There are however proposals that private personal use of the drug should not be an offence. The Liberal Democratic party adopted this as a resolution at its Spring conference in 2002. If a Bill is introduced into Parliament and has sufficient support, then there could be amendments to the Misuse of Drugs Act which legalises the use of cannabis in specified situations, but possibly still retaining the criminal offence of dealing. Following approval by both the House of Commons and the House of Lords and the Queen's signature, the Bill would become an Act and could be brought into force by Statutory Instrument on a specified date.

Decided cases

The other main source of law is the decisions of the courts. This source is known as case law, judge made law or the common law. The courts form a hierarchy with the highest court in this country being the Supreme Court (replacing the judicial House of Lords in October 2009). If the Supreme Court sets down a specific principle, known as a precedent, then this is binding on all courts in the country, except itself (i.e. the Supreme Court does not have to follow its own precedents). Following the Hillsborough football disaster, the House of Lords (as it was then) had to rule on whether it was lawful to withdraw artificial feeding from a patient in a persistent vegetative state (*Airedale NHS Trust v Bland [1993]*). It held that artificial feeding for Tony Bland could cease, on the basis that that was in his best interests. (This is considered in *Chapter 11*.)

Each decision of the courts is reported so that lawyers and judges can refer to the case and the principles it established, known as the *ratio decidendi,* can be applied to any matters in dispute.

If there is a dispute between a case and a statute the latter would take priority: judges have to follow an Act of Parliament. For example, in the Diane Pretty case, which is considered in *Chapter 2*, the House of Lords could not overrule the Suicide Act which made it a criminal offence for her husband to assist her to die. Had it thought that the Suicide Act was contrary to the European Convention on Human Rights (see below), then it could have referred it back to Parliament. It did not do this. Parliament can enact legislation which would overrule a principle established in the courts. If Jane (*Box 1.1*) were to be convicted for the offence of possession of cannabis, the judge would have considerable discretion over her punishment, from an absolute discharge to imprisonment. The court could not, however, overrule the Act of Parliament which made the possession of cannabis illegal.

Human Rights Act 1998

The Human Rights Act 1998 came into force in England, Wales and Northern Ireland on 2 October 2000 and on Devolution in Scotland. It incorporates the articles of the European Convention on Human Rights into our laws and is considered in *Chapter 2*.

Effect of the European Community

Since the UK signed the Treaty of Rome in 1972, the UK has become one of the member states of the European Community. The effect of this is that the UK is now subject to the laws made by the Council of Ministers and the European Commission. In addition secondary legislation of the European Community in the form of regulations is binding on the member states. Directives of the Community must be incorporated by Act of Parliament into the law of each member state. Appeals from UK courts on EC laws can be made to the European Court of Justice in Luxembourg which gives interpretations of the European laws. Their decisions are binding on the courts of member states.

Criminal laws and civil laws

A major distinction in the law of the UK is that between criminal laws and civil laws. The criminal law is considered in *Chapter 3* and civil law in *Chapter 4*. Some acts may be actionable as both a criminal offence and also a civil wrong. For example in *Chapter 6*, the action for trespass to the person is discussed. This action can be brought where treatment is given without the consent of the individual and in the absence of other factors which would be a defence to the action (e.g. acting in the best interests of a mentally incapacitated adult under the Mental Capacity Act 2005). A trespass may however also be a criminal act of assault and battery and there could be a prosecution in the criminal courts. It can be seen from this that there is not necessarily a moral difference between a crime and a civil wrong.

Legal personnel

Lawyers in this country are trained as solicitors or barristers. The former in the past have had direct dealings with clients and arranged with barristers (known as counsel) for the paperwork to be drafted and for representation of the client in court. They share a common foundation training: either a law degree or success in the Common Professional Examination and then would-be solicitors undertake practical training with a firm of solicitors, and take the Law Society's Part 2 examination, called the Legal Practice Course, whilst would-be barristers study for the Bar with the Council for Legal Education and are then 'called' to the bar after having dined on a specified number of occasions at one of the Inns of Court to which they must belong. A barrister who wishes to practise must then undertake pupillage where he or she is attached to a practising barrister. Senior barristers are eligible 'to take silk', i.e. they become Queen's Counsel (QC) appointed by the Lord Chancellor. Over recent years there have been considerable changes enabling solicitors to have wider opportunities to speak on behalf of clients in court and recently clients have been permitted to have direct access to a barrister. The likely result of all these developments may in the end be a single profession.

Legal Aid and conditional fees

Major changes have been made to the Legal Aid system under the Access to Justice Act 1999 (as amended by the Coroners and Justice Act 2009).

Part I of the Act provides for two new schemes, replacing the existing Legal Aid scheme, to secure the provision of publicly-funded legal services for people who need them. It establishes a Legal Services Commission to run the two schemes, and enables the Lord Chancellor to give the Commission orders, directions and guidance about how it should exercise its functions. It requires the Commission to establish, maintain and develop a Community Legal Service. The Community Legal Service fund replaces the Legal Aid fund in civil and family cases. The Commission is also responsible for a Criminal Defence Service, which replaces the current Legal Aid scheme in criminal cases. The new scheme is intended to ensure that people suspected or accused of a crime are properly represented, while securing better value for money than is possible under the Legal Aid scheme. The Legal Services Commission is empowered to secure these services through contracts with lawyers in private practice, or by providing them through salaried defenders (employed directly by the Commission or by non-profit-making organisations established for the purpose).

Part II of the Access to Justice Act 1999 makes changes to facilitate the private funding of litigation. A scheme known as 'no win, no fee' or conditional fee system has been introduced. By this system potential litigants can agree with lawyers terms on which they will be represented. Insurance cover is taken out to meet the expenses of witnesses and other costs arising in case the action is lost. The 1999 Act amends the law on conditional fee agreements between lawyers and their clients, in particular it allows the additional fees payable to a solicitor in a successful case in a no win no fee agreement, to be recovered from the other side. In a recent court decision the Court of Appeal has agreed that the costs of taking out insurance at a reasonable premium could be recovered from the losing party (*Callery v Gray; Russell v Pal Pak Corrugated Ltd* [2001]).

It is impossible in a work of this size to deal adequately with the complexities of the legal system and the procedures that are followed. The interested reader is therefore referred to the works in the list of further reading on p 177.

Ethics and law contrasted

One's ethics or moral standards derive from a variety of sources; religion, upbringing and personal experience all lead to a person's ethical values. In any democratic society one would hope that there would be a strong reciprocal relationship between the law and ethics. Therefore many civil and criminal wrongs would also be regarded as ethically wrong. However inevitably there are likely to be some gaps. For example in the situation in *Box 1.1* June may consider that she is morally right in obtaining cannabis to control her pain. After all what harm is she causing to anyone? Yet at the present time the Misuse of Drugs Act 1971 and the subsequent regulations makes it a criminal offence.

In this book we are concerned with the law and therefore there can be little discussion of ethical issues. However, in many of the situations we discuss there is also a moral or ethical perspective and the reader is referred to the further reading list for sources on ethics in healthcare for further discussion of this.

Codes of practice and conduct

Codes of practice and conduct are not in themselves 'laws'. They do however provide guidance for professional practice and could be used in evidence in civil or professional conduct proceedings that reasonable practice has not been followed. This is discussed further in *Chapter 5*.

Application of the law to the situation in *Box 1.1*

As the law stands at present Jane is guilty of a criminal offence. However, if she were to plead guilty to the offence it is hoped that any magistrate or judge sentencing her would take into account the mitigating circumstances and it may be that she could be given a conditional discharge.

Questions and exercises

1. Do you consider that the laws on cannabis should be changed to decriminalise its use?
2. To what extent do you consider that the criminal law and ethical principles should be identical?
3. Do you consider that barristers and solicitors should combine in a single legal profession?
4. Consider your own ethical principles. Are there any circumstances in which they do not accord 100% with the laws in this country?

References

Airedale NHS Trust v Bland [1993] 1 All ER 821

Callery v Gray; Russell v Pal Pak Corrugated Ltd TLR 18 July 2001

Dimond B (2008) *Legal Aspects of Nursing* (5th edn) London: Pearson

CHAPTER 2

Human rights

Box 2.1 Situation
Jane who suffered from MS was prosecuted for having cannabis in her possession. She pleaded not guilty and argued that since it had pain relieving properties she had a human right to use it and should not be guilty of a criminal offence.

Introduction

This country was a signatory of the European Convention in 1950 and accepted the articles on human rights. However the Convention was not incorporated into our law at that time. If a person considered his or her rights had been infringed then he or she would have to take the case to Strasbourg, where the European Court of Human Rights was sited, and to argue the case there. Parliament has now passed the Human Rights Act 1998. This came into force on 2 October 2000 for England, Wales and Northern Ireland (in Scotland the Act came into force earlier on Devolution). The Articles of the European Convention on Human Rights, which is set out in Schedule 1 to the Human Rights Act 1998 can be found in Appendix 1. The Act:

- requires all public authorities to implement the articles of the European Convention on Human Rights,
- gives a right to anyone who alleges that a public authority has failed to respect those rights to bring an action in the courts of this country, and
- enables judges who consider that legislation is incompatible with the Articles of the Convention to refer that legislation back to Parliament.

The duty to respect human rights as set out in the Articles is placed upon a public authority or organisation exercising functions of a public nature. This latter phrase received a narrow interpretation by the House of Lords (*YL v Birmingham City Council* [2007]) when it held, in a majority decision, that private care homes under contract with local authorities for the provision of places were not exercising functions of a public nature for the purposes of the Human Rights Act. The implications of this were that many thousands of

---

Box 2.2 The case of Diane Pretty

Diane Pretty was a terminally ill and incapacitated person suffering from motor neurone disease. She had minimum movement and was unable to attempt to commit suicide. She wished to die but would require assistance which her husband was prepared to give. She was mentally alert and wished to control the time and manner of her dying so as to avoid the suffering and indignity she would otherwise have to endure. The husband wished to have an undertaking from the Director of Public Prosecutions (DPP) that were he to aid and abet her suicide, he would not be prosecuted under Section 2(1) of the Suicide Act 1961 which makes it a criminal offence to aid and abet a suicide.

---

people being cared for in care homes would not be able to insist in law that their human rights were respected. As a consequence of the public outcry, Parliament has amended the law. Section 145 of the Health and Social Care Act 2008 provides for the provision of certain social care to be seen as a public function. Section 145 states that:

(1) A person ('P') who provides accommodation, together with nursing or personal care, in a care home for an individual under arrangements made with P under the relevant statutory provisions* is to be taken for the purposes of subsection (3)(b) of section 6 of the Human Rights Act 1998 (c. 42) (acts of public authorities) to be exercising a function of a public nature in doing so.

The House of Lords considered the Articles of the European Convention in the case of Diane Pretty (*Regina [Pretty] v Director of Public Prosecutions, Secretary of State for the Home Department intervening*). The facts of the case are set out in *Box 2.2*

It was argued on behalf of Diane Pretty that the provisions of the Suicide Act 1961 were incompatible with the European Convention on Human Rights. Articles 2, 3, 8, 9 and 14 were specifically identified as supporting her case.

Article 2: The right to life

It was argued that Article 2 protected the right to self-determination in relation to issues of life and death. It therefore recognised the individual's right to

---

* *The relevant statutory provisions means in relation to England and Wales Sections 21(1) (a) and 26 of the National Assistance Act 1948 (c. 29); in relation to Scotland, Section 12 or 13A of the Social Work (Scotland) Act 1968 (c. 49), and in relation to Northern Ireland, Articles 15 and 36 of the Health and Personal Social Services (Northern Ireland) Order 1972 (S.I. 1972/1265 (N.I. 14))*

choose whether or not to live and the state had a positive obligation to protect such a right as it had to protect the right to life.

The House of Lords however held that the thrust of the language of Article 2 reflected the sanctity attached to life, affording protection to the right to life and preventing the deliberate taking of life save in narrowly defined circumstances. The article could not be interpreted as conferring a right to die or to enlist the aid of another in bringing about one's own death. The argument put forward on behalf of Diane Pretty ignored two principles deeply embedded in English law:

- The distinction between taking one's own life by one's own act, permissible since suicide ceased to be a crime in 1961, and the taking of life through the intervention of help of a third party which continued to be proscribed. This principle was stated by the House of Lords in the Tony Bland case (*Airedale NHS Trust v Bland* [1993]).
- The distinction between the cessation of life-saving or prolonging treatment on the one hand and the taking of action lacking medical, therapeutic or palliative justification but intended solely to terminate life on the other hand (*J[re] [a minor] [wardship: medical treatment]* [1991]). This distinction proved the rationale for the decisions in Bland.

There was nothing to suggest that these two principles of English law were inconsistent with the rulings in the European Court of Human Rights in Strasbourg.

It was not enough for Mrs Pretty to show that the UK would not be acting inconsistently with the Convention if it were to permit assisted suicide, she had to go further and establish that the UK was in breach of the Convention by failing to permit it or would be so if it did not permit it. Such a contention was untenable.

Article 3: Prohibition of degrading and inhuman treatment

The House of Lords held that Article 3 required States to respect the physical and human integrity of individuals within their jurisdiction. There was nothing in Article 3 which bore on an individual's right to live or choose not to live. 'Treatment' should not be defined in an unrestricted or extravagant way. It could not be plausibly suggested that the Director of Public Prosecutions (DPP) or any other agent of the UK was inflicting the proscribed treatment on Mrs Pretty, whose suffering derived from her cruel disease. By no legitimate process of interpretation could the DPP's refusal of proleptic immunity from prosecution to Mr Pretty, if he committed a crime, be held to fall within the negative prohibition of Article 3.

The House of Lords also held that even if Article 3 was held to apply, there was no arguable breach of the negative prohibition in the article. It could not be said that the UK was under a positive obligation to ensure that a competent terminally ill person who wished but was unable to take his or her own life should be entitled to seek the assistance of another without that other being exposed to the risk of prosecution.

Article 8: Right to respect of private and family life

It was argued on behalf of Mrs Pretty that certain features of her case: her mental competence, the frightening prospect facing her, her willingness to commit suicide if she were able, the imminence of death, the absence of harm to anyone else, the absence of far-reaching implications if her application were granted and the blanket prohibition of Section 2(1) of the Suicide Act applied without taking account of particular cases, was wholly disproportionate and that the materials relied on did not justify it.

The House of Lords held that no cases decided in Strasbourg supported her contention and in fact her rights under Article 8 were not relevant to the case. Even if this was wrong, infringement was justifiable under Article 8.2. The decriminalising of assisted suicide had been reviewed several times (Criminal Law Revision Committee, 1980; Select Committee of the House of Lords, 1994) and change was unambiguously opposed. Assisted suicide and consensual killing were unlawful in all Convention countries except The Netherlands but even there Mr Pretty would be liable if he were to assist Mrs Pretty to take her own life.

Article 9: Freedom of thought

It was claimed for Mrs Pretty that her right to protection of freedom of thought, conscience and religion and the manifestation of religion or belief in worship, teaching, practice or observance had been violated. The House of Lords rejected this argument.

Article 14: Prohibition of discrimination

It was argued on Mrs Pretty's behalf that Section 2(1) of the Suicide Act discriminated against those who, like herself, could not, because of incapacity, take their own lives without assistance. The House of Lords rejected this claim. It held that the Strasbourg case decisions held that Article 14 was not autonomous but had effect only in relation to Convention rights. Therefore if none of the articles cited by Mrs Pretty gave her the right she claimed, then Article 14 would not assist her, even if she were able to establish that the effect of Section 2(1) of the Suicide Act was discriminatory. The criminal law could not in any event be criticised as discriminatory because it applied to all.

The Director of Public Prosecutions (DPP)

The DPP had argued that he had no power to grant the undertaking sought. The power to dispense with and suspend laws and their execution without parliamentary consent was denied to the Crown and its servants by the Bill of Rights 1699. Even if he did have power to give the undertaking sought he would have been very wrong to have done so here. He had no means of investigating the assertions made on Mrs Pretty's behalf; he had had no information at all concerning the means proposed for ending her life. No medical supervision was proposed. It would be a gross dereliction of the DPP's duty and a gross abuse of his power had he ventured to undertake that a crime yet to be committed would not lead to prosecution. The claim against him had to fail on that ground alone.

Outcome following the House of Lords case

Mr and Mrs Pretty were clearly disappointed with the decision by the House of Lords and took their case to the European Court of Human Rights in Strasbourg. On 29 April 2002 the European Court of Human Rights in Strasbourg ruled (*Pretty v UK [2002]*) that the UK Suicide Act (see *Chapter 11*), which made it a criminal offence to aid and abet a suicide, was not contrary to the European Convention on Human Rights. The Court stated:

> To seek to build into the law an exemption for those judged to be incapable of committing suicide would seriously undermine the protection of life, which the 1961 Suicide Act was intended to safeguard, and greatly increase the risk of abuse.

The case of Debbie Purdy

In 2009 Debbie Purdy (*R. [Purdy] v Director of Public Prosecutions [2009]*) challenged the uncertainty of the law on attempted suicide by seeking clarification of when a prosecution would be brought in relation to those who helped others end their lives. The case and the resulting guidelines from the Director of Public Prosecutions are discussed in *Chapter 11*.

Applying the Human Rights Convention to Jane's situation

Many of the arguments used on behalf of Diane Pretty could also be used on behalf of Jane (*Box 2.1*), yet probably with the same defeat. She might argue that since cannabis could relieve her pain, then the law making possession of cannabis a criminal offence is causing her to suffer inhuman and degrading treatment and punishment. Against this it could be argued that it is not the State that is causing her pain; it is her own illness and there are alternative ways of controlling the pain, other than the use of illegal substances. There has not to the author's knowledge been a case where a human rights argument has been successfully used in court to justify committing the offence of the possession of unlawful substances. However, the possibility that private use of cannabis may eventually be lawful may remedy Jane's situation.

Conclusion

The 2 October 2000 was feared by many NHS trusts, health professionals and lawyers as likely to lead to an avalanche of claims and law suits, but, like the millennium bug in the field of computers, this has not happened. What appears to have happened is that many litigants are adding a 'human rights' argument to their litigation. Thus a claim for compensation for negligence may be supported by arguing 'and in addition Article 3 of the Convention has been breached'. In general, the courts have taken a conservative attitude to the Human Rights Act 1998. However, there have been many successful cases and undoubtedly it is one of the most important and significant pieces of legislation of the last century in the UK. Even when human rights violation claims are defeated in the UK courts, the claimant can still apply to Strasbourg as the case of Mrs Pretty shows (although, as seen above, she lost). Absence of an effective system for pain management may be categorised as a breach of Article 3 of the European Convention.

Legal issues relating to a hospital or community wide pain management service are considered in *Chapter 17*.

References

Airedale NHS Trust v Bland [1993] 1 All ER 821

Criminal Law Revision Committee (1980) *14th Report*

J(re) (a minor)(wardship: medical treatment) [1991] Fam 33

Pretty v UK [2002] ECHR 427

Regina (Pretty) v Director of Public Prosecutions, Secretary of State for the Home Department intervening. TLR 5 December 2001; [2001] UKHL 61; [2001] 3 WLR 1598; [2002] 1 All ER 1

R (Purdy) v Director of Public Prosecutions TLR 24 February 2009

R (Purdy) v Director of Public Prosecutions. TLR 31 July 2009 HL

Select Committee of the House of Lords (1994) *Cmnd 7844*

YL v Birmingham City Council [2007] UKHL 22; The Times 21 June 2007

Criminal law

What is a crime?

There are laws that mostly derive from statutes, which create offences that can be followed by criminal proceedings in the form of a prosecution. An example of a statutory provision giving rise to criminal proceedings is the Misuse of Drugs Act 1971 which creates specific criminal offences in relation to controlled drugs which are divided into different schedules for the purpose of the criminal laws.

An example of case law that gives rise to criminal proceedings is the definition of murder, which was set out in a case in the 17th century.

Most of our criminal laws are enforced by prosecutions brought by the Crown Prosecution Service which was created in 1985. Other bodies also have powers to prosecute in specific cases, e.g. the Health and Safety Inspectorate, the National Society for the Prevention of Cruelty to Children, and Environmental Health Officers. There are other criminal laws such as those created by Local Authority powers known as by-laws which create local offences. There is also a right of an individual to bring a private prosecution, but this can be costly and of uncertain benefit.

Ingredients of a criminal offence

Whether the criminal offence originates in legislation (e.g. the Offences against the Person Act 1861) or case law (such as murder), there are two major elements in the definition of the offence: the physical acts – known as the *actus reus*; and the mental element – known as the *mens rea*. Both elements must be established beyond reasonable doubt in order to secure a conviction.

The *mens rea*, or mental element, includes all those elements that relate to the mind of the accused. The *actus reus* is everything else. There are some crimes where there is no requirement to show a mental element. For example, the sale of medicine by a person who was not qualified and while unsupervised by a pharmacist and which was contrary to Section 52 of the Medicines Act 1968 was once held to be a strict liability offence (*Pharmaceutical Society of Great Britain v Logan* [1982]). The law has now been changed. As a rule, however, there is a distaste for offences of strict liability, i.e. where there is no requirement for the prosecution to prove *mens rea*.

Criminal hearings

A prosecution is brought in relation to a charge of a criminal offence and heard in the criminal courts where the standard of proof is beyond reasonable doubt. Summary offences are heard in the Magistrates court and indictable offences (the more serious offences) in the Crown court, following committal proceedings in the Magistrates. Many offences are triable either way and the accused can opt for trial by jury. Currently there are Home Office plans to extend the number of offences that can only be heard by Magistrates. In the Magistrates court, the Magistrates decide if, on the facts, guilt has been established and if so, sentence the accused. They also have the power to remit the accused to the Crown court for sentencing by the Crown court judge. In the Crown court, the jury decides if the accused is guilty and if so the judge sentences the person convicted.

Criminal negligence

Gross negligence in professional practice may amount to the crime of manslaughter. For example, an anaesthetist failed to realise that during an operation a tube had become disconnected, as a result of which the patient died. He was prosecuted in the criminal courts and convicted of manslaughter (*R v Adomako* [1995]). There would also be liability on his employers in the civil courts for his negligence in causing the death of the patient. The Coroners and Justice Act 2009 has introduced several changes to the law on murder and manslaughter which are considered in *Chapter 11*.

The Law Commission (1996) recommended that the law should be changed to enable it to be made easier for corporations and statutory bodies to be prosecuted for manslaughter. As a consequence, the Corporate Manslaughter and Corporate Homicide Act 2007 was passed.

Corporate Manslaughter and Corporate Homicide Act 2007

The Act abolishes the common law offence of corporate manslaughter by gross negligence by an organisation and replaces it with statutory offences that can be committed by specified organisations if its activities are managed or organised in a way which (a) causes a person's death, and (b) amounts to a gross breach of a relevant duty of care owed by the organisation to the deceased. An organisation is guilty of an offence under this section only if the way in which its activities are managed or organised by its senior management is a substantial element in the breach of the duty of care. The organisations specified include 'corporations' and also the Department of Health. The duty of care is defined widely and includes duties to a detained patient, but excludes any duty of care owed by a public authority in respect of a decision as to matters of public policy (including in particular the allocation of public resources or the weighing of competing public interests). Duty of care also excludes emergency responses carried out by an NHS body or ambulance service. The jury determines if there has been a gross breach of the duty of care beyond reasonable doubt. On conviction the organisation can be fined, subjected to remedial order and required to publish details of the offence, the fine and the remedial action ordered. A prosecution under health and safety laws can proceed at the same time as a prosecution for corporate manslaughter. Individuals cannot be prosecuted under the Act, but they are liable to a common law prosecution for manslaughter and, if gross negligence which caused the death is established, can be convicted of manslaughter. (See the case of *R v Adomako* [1995] above.) Following conviction a company could be given an unlimited fine.

Accusatorial system

A feature of the legal system in this country is that it consists of one side with the responsibility of proving that the other side is at fault or guilty, or liable, of the wrong or crime alleged. This is known as an accusatorial system and it applies to both civil and criminal proceedings. In criminal cases the prosecution attempts to show beyond all reasonable doubt that the accused is guilty of the offence with which he or she is charged. The Magistrates, or the jury in the Crown court, determine whether the prosecution has succeeded in establishing the guilt of the accused, who is presumed innocent until proved guilty. In civil proceedings, the claimant (originally known as the plaintiff), i.e. the person bringing the action, has to establish on a balance of probability that there is negligence, trespass, nuisance or whatever civil wrong is alleged. In civil cases (apart from defamation) there is no jury and the judge has the responsibility of determining whether the plaintiff has succeeded in establishing the civil wrong.

The role of the judge or Magistrate is to chair the proceedings, intervening where necessary in the interests of justice, and advising on points of law and procedure.

The accusatorial system contrasts with a system of law which is known as inquisitorial where the judge plays a far more active role in determining the outcome. An example of an inquisitorial system in this country is the Coroner's court. Here the Coroner is responsible for deciding which witnesses would be relevant to answer to the questions that are placed before him by statute. Section 5 of the Coroners and Justice Act 2009 requires the coroner to ascertain:

- who the deceased was;
- how, when and where the deceased came by his or her death;
- the particulars (if any) required by the 1953 Act to be registered concerning the death.

In addition, under Section 5(2) where necessary in order to avoid a breach of any Convention rights (within the meaning of the Human Rights Act 1998 [c. 42]), the purpose mentioned in subsection (1)(b) is to be read as including the purpose of ascertaining in what circumstances the deceased came by his or her death.

The Coroner asks the witnesses questions in court and decides who else can ask questions and what they can ask. As a result of this 'inquisition', the Coroner or a jury, if one is used, determine the cause of death.

Application of the law to the situation in *Box 3.1*

Alsana will have to face the consequences of her crime, no matter how noble her objective. This would be taken into account in determining the sentence, not of her guilt or innocence. At the present time she would have the right to elect jury trial. She would face committal proceedings before the Magistrates and if committed to the Crown court, would plead to the charge. If she pleaded not guilty she would then face a trial before a jury.

Conclusions

There have been several cases where health professionals have been prosecuted in relation to their care of the patient, such as those of Dr Shipman who was found guilty of the murder of 15 patients using morphine, Dr Cox who was found guilty of attempted murder when he injected a patient who was in the terminal stages of rheumatoid arthritis with potassium chloride, and Dr Bodkin Adams who was found not guilty of killing a patient in an Eastbourne nursing home. These are considered in *Chapter 11*.

References

Law Commission (1996) *No 237 Legislating the Criminal Code: Involuntary Manslaughter*. London: HMSO

Pharmaceutical Society of Great Britain v Logan [1982] Crim. LR 443

R v Adomako [1995] 1 AC 171; [1994] 3 All ER 79 HL TLR July 4 (1994)

CHAPTER 4

Negligence

> **Box 4.1 Situation**
>
> May was administering medication for pain relief to a child and accidentally gave 10 times the prescribed dose. The child suffered a cardiac arrest and May immediately sought help and admitted her mistake. Unfortunately the child died.

Civil laws

These are laws (both statutory and case law) which enable citizens to claim remedies against other citizens or organisations as a result of a civil wrong. A large group of civil wrongs are known as torts, of which negligence is the main one, but the group also includes action for breach of statutory duty, nuisance, and defamation. Actions for breach of contract are not included in the definition of tort. An example of a statute that can give rise to civil action is the Congenital Disabilities Act 1976 which gives a child, who is born alive, the right to sue in respect of negligence which led to him or her suffering from a congenital defect. An example of a case where an application was made to the High Court is that of Diane Pretty which is discussed in *Chapter 2*. In this chapter we consider the law of negligence and how it applies to pain management practitioners.

Elements of a negligence action

A claimant alleging that negligence has occurred and seeking compensation in respect of harm caused by that negligence would have to establish the following elements:

* that a duty of care was owed by the defendant or its employees in relation to the person who has suffered harm,
* that there was a reasonably foreseeable breach of this duty,
* which caused reasonably foreseeable harm,
* that was recognised in law as subject to compensation.

Duty of care

Case law has laid down that a duty of care is owed to those persons who are so directly affected by another's acts that they ought reasonably to be considered as being so affected when the defendant is directing his mind to the acts or omissions that are called in question (see *Donoghue v Stevenson* [1932]). However the law does not require a person to volunteer to assist another, unless there is an existing duty of care. So the law does not require a health professional to volunteer to assist at a road accident, although the codes of professional conduct of specific health professionals may require such Good Samaritan acts. For example, the NMC Code of 2004 paragraph 8.5 made it explicit that the nurse had a professional duty to provide care. In the 2008 edition of the Code such a duty is no longer set out explicitly but could be inferred from the words, 'You must uphold the reputation of your profession at all times'.

Breach of the duty of care

In order to establish if there has been a breach of the duty of care it is essential to establish what standard should have been followed. The courts have used what has become known as the Bolam Test to determine the standard to be expected of a health professional in a specific situation. This derives from case of *Bolam v Friern Hospital Management Committee* [1957]. The test was applied in the case of a obstetrician who was alleged to have pulled too long and too hard in a forceps delivery. The House of Lords held that on the facts a breach of the duty of care had not been established and stated as follows:

> *When you get a situation which involves the use of some special skill or competence, then the test as to whether there has been negligence or not is ... the standard of the ordinary skilled man exercising and professing to have that special skill. If a surgeon failed to measure up to that in any respect ('clinical judgement' or otherwise) he had been negligent and should be so adjudged.*
>
> *Whitehouse v Jordan* [1981]

Expert evidence is required to establish what would be the reasonable standard of care in the circumstances of the case and whether, on the facts, that was followed. Experts are required to give 'responsible, reasonable and respectable opinions relating to the facts of the case' (*Bolitho v City and Hackney Health Authority* [1997]) and the recent reforms in civil proceedings following from the report of Lord Woolf recommend that the parties should agree on the experts to give evidence to the court.

Increasingly, guidelines from such bodies as the National Institute of Health and Clinical Excellence and the National Service Frameworks are likely to be incorporated in NHS trust procedures and protocols setting out the reasonable standard of acceptable clinical practice. However there may still be occasions where the specific circumstances of the patient are such that the procedures are not entirely appropriate and so deviations from it are justified. The House of Lords stated in the Maynard case (*Maynard v W. Midlands RHA* [1984]) that:

...it was not sufficient to establish negligence for the claimant to show that there was a body of competent professional opinion that considered that the decision had been wrong if there was also a body of equally competent professional opinion that supported the decision as having been reasonable in the circumstances.

Causation

Failure to establish a causal link between the breach of the duty of care and the harm that was suffered would mean that the claim for compensation would not succeed in court. In one case (*Kay v Ayrshire and Arran Health Board* [1987]) a child suffering from meningitis was given 300 000 units of penicillin instead of 10 000 units. The mistake was discovered and remedial action taken. The health authority admitted liability and made an offer to the parents for the additional pain and suffering that the negligence caused the boy. However, the parents argued that the overdose had caused the boy to become deaf and they rejected the Board's offer. The House of Lords held that the parents had not established the causal link between the overdose and the deafness and thus that the boy was not entitled to the larger amount. It is a well-known fact that meningitis itself can cause deafness.

Harm

The claimant must establish that he or she has suffered harm. Harm recognised by the courts as subject to compensation includes personal injury and death and loss or damage to property. Specific rules apply where it is claimed that post-traumatic stress has been caused (*McLoughlin v O'Brian* [1982]; *Alcock v Chief Constable S Yorks Police* [1992]; *White and others v Chief Constable of the South Yorkshire Police and others* [1999]).

Quantum or level of compensation

Occasionally it might be accepted by a defendant that it is liable, but the amount of compensation payable may be disputed. Where a death has occurred, there is a statutory payment of £11 800 known as a bereavement allowance and this would be payable in respect of a person without dependants. Where there are dependants, however, they could claim for the loss of their dependency.

The headings for compensation include general damages which cannot easily be calculated in financial terms such as pain suffering and loss of amenity, and special damages which include sums already paid out and those which can be more closely calculated such as interest, past care, accommodation, future care, claimant's loss of earnings, other future expenses and education

Vicarious liability

In practice the claimant would bring an action against the employer and would have to show that there was negligence caused by an employee who was acting in the course of employment. The employer would then be vicariously liable for the employee's negligence and would have to pay the compensation. Those health practitioners who are self-employed cannot rely on vicarious liability and would have to have their own insurance cover.

Application of the law to the situation in *Box 4.1*

In a situation such as *Box 4.1* the death would be reported to the coroner and subsequently there may well be criminal investigations to establish whether May was guilty of a criminal offence (see *Chapter 3*). If civil proceedings were to be brought May clearly has a duty of care to her patient; it would appear difficult to argue that a nurse who failed to administer what was correctly prescribed could be anything other than in breach of the duty of care she owed to the patient. The boy's parents would also have to show that the death occurred as a result of the breach of duty of care by May. A post mortem may be required to establish if there was causation between the overdose and the death. It is unlikely that May would have to pay compensation herself, since her employer would be vicariously liable for her negligence. There is a legal right of indemnity by the employer against a negligent employee to recover the compensation paid out, but an NHS trust is unlikely to claim this indemnity from May successfully.

The future

In spite of the significant reforms introduced by Lord Woolf in civil proceedings, bringing a claim for compensation in the civil courts is still seen as a slow, expensive and cumbersome procedure. In addition the cost of litigation to the NHS is climbing and shows no signs of decreasing. In September 2007 it was revealed that current claims against the NHS for negligence handled by the NHS Litigation Authority amounted to almost £4.5 billion, of which £3.3 billion related to incidents alleging oxygen starvation at birth. In the decade ending in 2008 there were 1179 clinical negligence claims relating to cancer treatment leading to £47 million paid out in compensation and claims of £50 million still outstanding (Rose, 2008). In the light of a report by the National Audit Office in 2001 on handling clinical negligence claims in England, the Department of Health (2001) proposed a new compensation scheme. *Making amends* was published in 2003 and proposed a new statutory scheme for compensation for the NHS. The NHS Redress Act 2006, which gives power to the Secretary of State to establish schemes for compensation operating alongside the current civil proceedings, has still to be brought into force.

Questions and exercises

1. What are your views on the introduction of a no-fault liability scheme for negligence in healthcare?
2. Do you consider that the employer's right of indemnity against the negligent employee should be exercised in the NHS?
3. How do you think that mediation would work in claims for compensation for clinical negligence?

References

Alcock v Chief Constable S. Yorks. Police [1992] 2 AC 310 HL

Bolam v Friern Barnet HMC [1957] 2 All ER 118

Bolitho v City and Hackney Health Authority [1997] 3 WLR 115

Department of Health (2001) *Press release 2001/0313 New Clinical Compensation Scheme for the NHS*. London: HMSO

Department of Health (2003) *Making amends: A consultation paper setting out proposals for reforming the approach to clinical negligence in the NHS*. London: Department of Health

Donoghue v Stevenson [1932] AC 562

Kay v Ayrshire and Arran Health Board [1987] 2 All ER 417

Maynard v W. Midlands RHA [1984] 1 WLR 634

McLoughlin v O'Brian [1982] 2 All ER 298

National Audit Office (2001) *Handling clinical negligence claims in England. Report of the Comptroller and Auditor General House of Commons Session 2000–2001*. National Audit Office

Nursing and Midwifery Council (2004, revised 2008) *Code of Professional Conduct: Standards for performance, conduct and ethics*. London: NMC

Rose D (2008) £100 million payouts for cancer negligence *The Times* 10 March

Whitehouse v Jordan [1981] 1 All ER 267

White and others v Chief Constable of the South Yorkshire Police and others
   [1999] 1 All ER 1

CHAPTER 5

Professional registration

> ## Box 5.1 Situation
> Chris, a physiotherapist specialising in back disorders, was caring for a patient with a chronic back pain. He was manipulating the patient's back when the patient screamed. It was subsequently established that Chris appeared to have caused serious injury to the patient's back. The patient wants to have Chris struck off the state registered list.

Introduction

Significant changes came into effect in April 2002 in respect of nurses, midwives, health visitors and all those professions previously described as 'professions supplementary to medicine'. Two new registration bodies: the Nursing and Midwifery Council (NMC) and the Health Professions Council (HPC) replaced the former United Kingdom Central Council for Nursing Midwifery and Health Visiting (UKCC) and the Council for the Professions Supplementary to Medicine (CPSM), respectively. Provision was also made in the NHS Reform and Healthcare Professions Act for the establishment of a Council for the Regulation of Healthcare Professions (now known as the Council for Healthcare Regulatory Excellence). This latter body is intended to oversee the operation of the NMC, the HPC, the General Medical Council, the General Dental Council and other health professionals' regulatory bodies.

The scope of the professional registration bodies

The main function of the registration bodies is to protect the public by maintaining a register of persons who have been assessed as competent practitioners and to ensure that any practitioner whose fitness to practise is brought into question is investigated and, if necessary, a conduct or health committee hearing is held. The ultimate sanction is removal from the register.

NMC and HPC

These organisations were established in April 2002 having existed in shadow form for almost a year before. Their basic functions are laid down in the Health Act 1999 and the detailed rules and regulations which apply to them are set out in statutory instruments (Nursing and Midwifery Order, 2001; Statutory Instrument, 2002; Health Professions Order, 2001).

The functions of the NMC and the HPC which, under Schedule 3 paragraph 8(2) of the Health Act 1999, cannot be delegated to any other body are shown in *Box 5.2.*

Box 5.2. Functions of the NMC and HPC

- Keeping the register of members admitted to practice
- Determining the standards of education and training for admission to practice
- Giving advice about standards of conduct and performance
- Administering procedures (including making rules) relating to misconduct, unfitness to practise and similar matters

---

Codes of professional practice

All registration bodies are expected to establish codes of professional conduct for their registered practitioners. These codes are not in themselves law, but breach of the code could be used as evidence in professional fitness to practice hearings. A new Code of Professional Conduct for nurses, midwives and health visitors was published by the NMC in 2008.

Definition of professional misconduct

In the past health professionals have had a variety of definitions of professional misconduct depending on their specific profession. For example those practitioners formerly registered with the CPSM could be found guilty of 'infamous conduct', whereas nurses, midwives and health visitors could face professional conduct proceedings for 'conduct unworthy of a nurse, midwife or health visitor'.

Under paragraph 9 of the Health Professions Council (Conduct and Competence Committee) Procedure Rules 2003, where the Committee has found that the health professional has failed to comply with the standards of conduct, performance and ethics established by the Council under article 21(1)(a) of the Health Professions Order 2001, the Committee may take that failure into account but such failure shall not be taken of itself to establish that the fitness to practise of the health professional is impaired.

Progress of a complaint

The complaint against the physiotherapist in *Box 5.1* would be reported to the Investigating Committee of the HPC. This is one of the statutory committees that the Health Professions Council is required to establish and they are known as Practice Committees. The others are the Conduct and Competence Committee and the Health Committee.

The Health Professions Order Article 22 (as amended) applies where an allegation is made against a registered person to the effect that:

(a) His fitness to practice is impaired by reason of:
    (i)   misconduct
    (ii) lack of competence
    (iii) a conviction or caution in the UK for a criminal offence; or a conviction elsewhere for an offence, which, if committed in England and Wales, would constitute a criminal offence,
    (iv) his physical or mental health, or
    (v) a determination by a body in the UK responsible under any enactment for the regulation of a health or social care profession to the effect that he is unfit to practise that profession, or a determination by a licensing body elsewhere to the same effect;
    (vi) the Independent Barring Board including the person in a barred list (within the meaning of the Safeguarding Vulnerable Groups Act 2006 or the Safeguarding Vulnerable groups (Northern Ireland) Order 2007), or
    (vii) the Scottish Ministers, including the person in the children's list or the adults' list (within the meaning of the Protection of Vulnerable Groups (Scotland) Act 2007).
(b) An entry in the register relating to him has been fraudulently procured or incorrectly made.

A procedure is laid down for dealing with such allegations. Where an allegation is made under (b) the Council must refer it to the Investigating Committee. All other allegations are to be referred to Screeners or a Practice Committee. Screeners are to be appointed by rules made by Council and can be members of the Council or its Committees, other than a Practice Committee

Articles 23 and 24 of the Health Professions Order cover the function and appointment of Screeners.

Under Article 26 the Investigating Committee shall investigate any allegation referred under Article 22 or 24. The procedure to be followed is set out.

Article 27 sets out the procedure to be followed by the Conduct and Competence Committee. After consultation with the other Practice Committees, the Conduct and Competence Committee shall

(a) delete, Health Care & Ass. Profs (Misc Amdts & Prac Psychs) Order 2009, Sch. 2, para 7
(b) consider:
    (i) any allegation referred to it by the Council, Screeners, the Investigating Committee or the Health Committee, and
    (ii) any application for restoration referred to it by the Registrar.

Under Article 28 the Health Committee shall consider any allegation referred to it by the Council, Screeners, the Investigating Committee or the Conduct and Competence Committee and any application for restoration referred to it by the Registrar.

Article 29 sets out the orders that can be made by the Health Committee and the Conduct and Competence Committee.

Article 31 covers interim orders which can be made by a Practice Committee to suspend a person's registration in specified circumstances.

Article 32 sets out the Procedural rules for an investigation of allegations.

Article 33 covers the provisions for restoration to the register of persons who have been struck off.

Article 34 covers the appointment of legal assessors. Legal assessors have the general function of giving advice to Screeners, the statutory committees or the Registrar on questions of law arising in connection with any matter which the Registrar of the Committee or Screeners are considering. Other functions can be given to the legal assessors by rules made by the Council

Article 35 covers the appointment of medical assessors to give advice to the same persons or committees as legal assessors.

Article 36 covers the appointment of registered professionals as registrant assessors with the function of giving advice on professional practice.

Civil standards of proof

The White Paper *Trust, Assurance and Safety – the Regulation of Health Professionals in the 21st Century* set out the Government's plan for modernising professional regulation to ensure that confidence in healthcare professionals will remain. Some of the recommendations were included in the Health and Social Care Act 2008. Section 112 of that Act introduced the civil standard of proof into fitness to practice proceedings of the regulatory bodies. This means that evidence of misconduct has to be established on a balance of probabilities rather than beyond reasonable doubt. The result is that it is now easier to find a case against a health professional established and thus provide better protection for the public. The NMC makes the comment that:

The move to the civil standard of proof does not mean that FtP [fitness to practise] hearings will be treated with any less seriousness; panels will continue to treat all allegations with the same level of gravity and expertise.

The NMC has 193 fitness to practise panelists, and is still recruiting more. All panellists will receive expert and practical training in how to apply the civil standard of proof from a legal firm.

Application of the law to the situation in *Box 5.1*

If Chris is employed, his employer may be sued by the patient for its vicarious liability for any harm caused by negligence by Chris (see *Chapter 4*). If he is self-employed, he may well face personal action against him. In addition the patient is indicating that he is to be reported to the Health Professions Council (HPC). If a complaint were to be made against Chris to the HPC (and a complaint against a nurse, midwife or health visitor would follow a similar path but to the Nursing and Midwifery Council), it would be investigated by the Investigating Committee and the procedure outlined above would be followed. Chris would have to be shown to be unfit to practise on a balance of probabilities, the civil standard of proof. Ultimately Chris faces the possibility of being removed from the register.

Conclusion

There is every likelihood that following the initial investigation Chris would face a hearing before the Conduct and Competence Committee with the possibility of being struck off from the HPC register. If he were not struck off, the complainant could complain to the new Council for Healthcare Regulatory Excellence which could apply to the High Court on the grounds that the regulatory body had dealt unduly leniently with an allegation of unfitness to practise. Additional powers were given to the Council for Healthcare Regulatory Excellence in 2009 to ensure that the public has greater protection from those healthcare professionals who are found to be unfit to practice.

Questions and exercises

1. To what extent do you consider that the public is adequately protected from practitioners who are not fit to practise?
2. How do you consider professional misconduct should be defined?
3. Examine the role of the Council for Healthcare Regulatory Excellence. Do you consider that it fulfils a useful purpose? Reference can be made to its website (www.chre.org.uk).

References

Health Professions Order 2001 SI 2002 No 254

Nursing and Midwifery Order 2001 Statutory Instrument 2002 No 253

Nursing and Midwifery Council (2008) *The Code. Standards of conduct, performance and ethics for nurses and midwives*. London: NMC

CHAPTER 6

Consent: Adults

> **Box 6.1 Situation**
>
> Julius was a Buddhist who led a very spartan and austere life. He was in the terminal stages of cancer of the pancreas and was in acute pain. However he was refusing any medication for pain relief. He was visited by a Marie Curie nurse from the local hospice who found it difficult to assist him when he was refusing the basic help which she could provide. She wondered if he could be forced to have medication for his pain. She was aware that his family was very distressed on his account.

The law of trespass to the person

Two legal actions can arise in relation to consent. The first is an action for trespass to the person, where there is no consent to the touching of another person or other legal justification, or there has been fraud or duress in obtaining the consent. In this action, harm need not be proved: merely the touching or apprehension of touching. Trespass to the person includes both battery (the actual touching of the person) and assault (the apprehension of the touching) Battery and assault are also criminal offences, but here we are considering them as civil wrongs. The other action that can arise in relation to consent is one of negligence where the person has not been informed of significant information. In this action the claimant would have to prove that the harm that has been suffered would not have been suffered if the information had been given. (This is considered in *Chapter 10*.)

The basic principle of law is that no mentally competent adult person can be treated, whatever the motive of the defendant, without their consent or statutory justification (for example, the Mental Health Act 1983). Reference can be made to the author's book on consent to treatment (Dimond, 2009).

Defences to an action for trespass to the person

The main defences to an action for trespass to the person are consent by a mentally capacitated person, acting in the best interests of a mentally incapacitated person under the provisions of the Mental Capacity Act 2005 and statutory justification such as the Mental Health Act 1983. In this chapter consent will be considered; acting on behalf of a mentally incapacitated person is considered in *Chapter 8*. The law relating to consent and children is considered in *Chapter 7*.

Consent

The main defence to an action for trespass to the person is that the person had given their consent to what would otherwise have been a trespass. The consent must have been given by a mentally competent person, voluntarily without duress or fraud and with the knowledge of what was proposed.

Guidance has been provided by the Department of Health on consent, which can be accessed via the Internet and is intended to be updated on a regular basis (Department of Health, 2001a).

Evidence of consent

Consent can be given by non-verbal behaviour, which implies agreement with the intended action (such as rolling up a sleeve for an injection or blood pressure reading to take place) or by word of mouth or in writing. Clearly if there is a dispute then consent in writing is the preferred evidence that consent was given, but the signature on the form should not be seen as the consent itself, but evidence, following a process of communication between health professional and patient, that the patient understands what is proposed and is giving his or her consent.

Forms have been issued by the Department of Health (2001b) as part of its Good Practice in Consent implementation guide, replacing those issued by the NHS Management Executive in 1990 and updated in 1992. The recommended forms can be used by any health professional.

Mentally competent adult

To be valid the consent must have been given by a mentally competent adult (for children see *Chapter 7*). There is a statutory presumption set by the Mental Capacity Act 2005 that a person over 16 years is presumed to have the requisite mental capacity but this presumption can be rebutted on a balance of probabilities. (See *Chapter 8* for the principles set down in the Mental Capacity Act 2005.)

Competence is a question of fact and applies to each specific decision to be made. It is possible for a person to have the requisite capacity to make one decision but not another.

In a case (*C [re]* [1994]) involving a Broadmoor patient, a chronic schizophrenic, who was refusing to have an amputation of his leg (even though he was warned that gangrene had set in and he could die without the amputation), the judge laid down three tests of capacity as follows:

• Could the patient comprehend and retain the necessary information?
• Was he able to believe it?
• Was he able to weigh the information, balancing risks and needs, so as to arrive at a choice?

Applying these tests to the Broadmoor patient, the judge decided that the patient did have the mental capacity to refuse and the judge issued an injunction to restrain any person amputating his leg without his consent.

The Mental Capacity Act 2005 has provided a statutory definition of mental incapacity. It is a two-fold test used at the time the decision is to be made. Firstly it must be established that a person is suffering from an impairment of, or a disturbance in the functioning of, the mind or brain. Secondly it must be shown that as a consequence of this impairment or disturbance, the person is unable to make a decision for himself in relation to the matter. Being unable to make a decision means that he is unable to

• understand the information relevant to the decision,
• retain that information,
• use or weigh that information as part of the process of making the decision, or
• communicate his decision (whether by talking, using sign language or any other means).

It does not matter whether the impairment or disturbance is permanent or temporary.

The Mental Capacity Act 2005 states that a lack of capacity cannot be established merely by reference to (a) a person's age or appearance, or (b) a condition of his, or an aspect of his behaviour, which might lead others to make unjustified assumptions about his capacity.

Superficial assumptions cannot therefore be the basis of a decision on whether or not a person has the requisite mental capacity.

Refusal

Once it is decided that the patient does have the mental capacity to give or refuse consent then the patient can refuse even life-saving treatment for a good reason, a bad reason or no reason at all (*MB (re) [an adult: medical treatment]* [1997]). The Court of Appeal has laid down guidance for applying to the court if there is a doubt over the mental capacity of the patient who is refusing life saving treatment (*St George's Healthcare NHS Trust v S; R v Collins ex parte S*

[1998]). In the case of *B (re)* [2002], the President of the Family Division stated that a mentally competent patient could ask for her ventilator to be switched off and that it was a trespass to her person to treat her without her consent. (See *Chapter 11* for further discussion of this case.)

Where a competent patient lays down in advance what he or she would not wish to happen at a later time – known as a living will or an advance decision or advance refusal – then this would be binding on health professionals. This is considered in *Chapter 9*.

Application of the law to the situation of Julius

The key issue in the situation in *Box 6.1* is the capacity of Julius. If he has the mental capacity then he has the right in law to make his own decisions and can refuse pain relief. Even if this is difficult for his family and his nurse to accept, it is his right. If there is concern as to whether he does have the mental capacity to refuse then an application could be made to court to establish whether he lacks the requisite mental capacity, in which case treatment could be given to him in his best interests. This is considered in *Chapter 8*. In *Chapter 9* on advance decisions, there is a discussion on whether an advance decision could apply to basic care such as pain relief and oral nutrition and hydration.

Questions and exercises

1. Do you consider that there should be any exceptions, such as pain relief, which should be made to the right of a mentally competent person to refuse treatment?
2. Examine your processes of obtaining consent. To what extent do you consider that they are sufficiently vigorous for you to defend an action for trespass to the person?
3. Define the circumstances in which you consider evidence in writing of the patient's consent to treatment should be obtained.

References

B (re) (consent to treatment: capacity) TLR 26 March 2002

C (re) (adult: refusal of medical treatment) Family Division [1994] 1 All ER 819

Department of Health (2001a) *Reference Guide to Consent for Examination or Treatment*. London: Department of Health. Available from: www. doh.gov. uk/consent

Department of Health (2001b) *Good Practice in Consent Implementation Guide*. London: Department of Health

Dimond B (2009) *Legal Aspects of Consent to Treatment* (2nd edn) London: Quay Books

MB (re) (an adult: medical treatment) [1997] 2 FLR 426

St George's Healthcare NHS Trust v S [1998] 44 BMLR 160 CA

R v Collins ex parte S [1998] 44 BMLR 160 CA

CHAPTER 7

Consent: Children

Box 7.1 Situation

Avril was 12 years old and seriously ill with cystic fibrosis. She knew that her lungs were severely damaged following constant chest infections and had been placed on a list for a lung transplant. She felt that she would prefer to die rather than put up with the pain, discomfort and suffering and had started refusing her physiotherapy and intravenous antibiotics. Her parents wanted her to continue to have active treatment so that she would be fit for a lung transplant which could revolutionise her life. What is the law?

Young persons aged 16 and 17 years

Consent by a 16- and 17-year-old

These young persons have a statutory right to give consent under the Family Law Reform Act 1969 Section 8. Consent can be given for surgical, medical and dental treatment and the definition of treatment covers any procedure undertaken for the purposes of diagnosis and any ancillary procedures such as administration of anaesthetic.

The parents also have the right to give consent on behalf of the 16- and 17-year-old. This is preserved by Section 8(3) of the Family Law Reform Act 1969. Where there is a clash between the parent and the minor, the professional would normally follow the wishes of the minor. However, much depends upon the circumstances.

Refusal by a 16- and 17-year-old

In the case of *W (re)* [1992], a 16-year-old who suffered from anorexia who refused to go to a specialist unit for treatment, the courts decided that she could be compelled to go against her wishes since it was in her best interests to receive treatment. The Court of Appeal held that the refusal of a minor should only be overruled in extreme circumstances where it was a life and death matter. However this decision was made before the Human Rights Act 1998 became part of English law on 2 October 2000 (see *Chapter 2* and *Appendix 1*).

It could be argued that failure to recognise the right of a young person to refuse treatment was a breach of Article 3 and his or her right not to be treated in an inhuman or degrading way. If, for example, W had been a Jehovah's Witness and had refused blood in a life-saving situation, then to overrule the refusal could have been seen as a violation of Article 3 and also Article 9 (freedom of thought, religion and practice). The point has yet to be considered by the House of Lords.

A mentally incapacitated 16- and 17-year-old

In the case of *B (re)* [1987] the House of Lords laid down the principles for decision making on behalf of a mentally incapacitated 17-year-old girl (see *Box 7.2*)

Box 7.2 Case Re B

A 17-year-old girl (who later became known as Jeanette) who had a mental age of five or six years was in the care of the local authority. It was established that she would have no understanding of sexual intercourse, pregnancy, and birth. The local authority applied for her to be made a ward of court and for leave to be given for the operation of sterilisation to be carried out.

The House of Lords held that the paramount consideration for the exercise of its wardship jurisdiction was the welfare and best interests of the child. The Court held that it was in the best interests of the minor for the sterilisation to proceed and permission was given for the operation to take place.

Since the Mental Capacity Act 2005 came into force, the Court of Protection hears cases relating to young persons over 16 years. Disputes relating to the mental capacity of a person aged 16 or 17 years could be heard either by the Court of Protection applying the Mental Capacity Act 2005 or by the Family Courts applying the Children Act 1989. Under Section 21 of the Mental Capacity Act 2005 the Court of Protection has the power in certain circumstances to transfer cases concerning children to a court that has jurisdiction under the Children Act 1989. In addition a case started in a court having jurisdiction under the Children Act 1989 can be transferred to the Court of Protection.

The child under 16 years

Whilst children under the age of 16 years do not have a statutory right to consent to treatment, the right to give consent at common law (i.e. judge-made law) was recognised by the House of Lords in the Gillick case (*Gillick v. W. Norfolk and Wisbech Area Health Authority* [1986]).

If a child has the maturity to understand the nature, purpose, and likely effects of any proposed treatment, then he or she could give a valid consent without the involvement of the parents. Whilst the Gillick case itself was concerned with family planning and treatment, the principle applies to other forms of treatment and to boys as well as girls. The principle that the ascertainable wishes and feelings of the child concerned (considered in the light of his or her age and understanding) should also be taken into account is also stated in the Children Act 1989 Section 1(3)(a) as one of the factors to which the court shall have regard in determining what if any orders should be made or varied.

Parents can also give consent to treatment on behalf of their children up to the age of 18 years. However such treatment must be in the best interests of the child. Persons who do not have parental responsibilities also have power under the Children Act 1989 Section 3(5), which enables a person who (a) does not have parental responsibility for a particular child, but (b) has care of the child to do what is reasonable in all the circumstances of the case for the purposes of safeguarding or promoting the child's welfare.

Parental refusal to give consent

If the parent or guardian of a minor under the age of 18 refused to give consent to treatment which was necessary in the best interests of the minor, the doctor could act out of necessity in the best interests of the minor according to the principle set out in *F (re)* (see *Chapter 8*). Alternatively the authority of the court could be sought for treatment to proceed against the parents' wishes. Should the parents fail to give consent to essential treatment or arrange for the treatment to take place, they can face prosecution in the event of harm befalling the child. For example, a Rastafarian couple who had refused on religious grounds to allow their diabetic daughter who was nine years old to be given insulin were convicted of manslaughter on 28 October 1993 in Nottingham. The father was given a sentence of imprisonment and the mother a suspended sentence (*The Times*, 29 October 1993).

Application of the law to the situation in *Box 7.1*

Avril is 12 years old and refusing life-saving treatment. Whilst she does not believe that she is likely to survive and receive a transplant, her parents clearly see this as a realistic possibility. Much depends upon her prognosis. It may be that she has become so ill that she would not have the physical capacity to survive a transplant operation. In this case it may well be in her best interests to be given palliative care to relieve her pain and discomfort but not active interventions. Such a decision needs to be discussed by the multidisciplinary team and Avril's parents and also, according to her mental capacity, Avril could be involved in the discussions. There will be situations where a child of even quite a young age has the mental capacity to understand the prognosis and take an active role in the decisions to be made. Ultimately if Avril does not have the mental capacity to make the decision, then the doctors caring for her would have to determine, in the light of her prognosis, what was in her best interests. In the event of a dispute between parents and clinicians, there would be a referral to court. There are very few cases where the courts have supported parents against the clinicians. In one case (*C [re] [a minor] [medical treatment: refusal of parental consent]* [1997]) parents refused to give consent to a liver transplant being carried out on their toddler. The Court of Appeal held that in the very specific circumstances of the case (the parents lived abroad and as health professionals they believed the transplant not to be in the best interests of the child) the transplant would not be ordered against their wishes.

Questions and exercises

1. What criteria would you use to decide if a young child had the capacity to give consent to treatment?
2. In what circumstances do you consider that a young person of 16 or 17 years of age should be able to refuse life-saving treatment?
3. In what circumstances do you consider that a parent should have the power to overrule a refusal to have necessary treatment by a child?

References

B (re) (a minor) (wardship: sterilisation) [1987] 2 All ER 206

C (re) (a minor) (medical treatment: refusal of parental consent) [1997] 8 Med LR 166 CA

Gillick v W Norfolk and Wisbech Area Health Authority [1986] 1 AC 112

W (re) (a minor)(medical treatment) 1992 4 All ER 627

CHAPTER 8

Consent: Mentally incapacitated adults

Box 8.1 Situation

Julie suffers from Alzheimer's disease and is in the terminal stages of lung cancer. She is intermittently competent and extremely aggressive towards her carers. She has been transferred from her family home where her daughter was caring for her to a hospice. The staff are uncertain of the extent to which they can compel her to have her medication, some of which is for pain relief.

Introduction

In *Chapter 6* the law relating to consent by a mentally capacitated adult was considered and it was stated that if a person had the mental capacity to make decisions on treatment, then he or she could refuse even life-saving treatment (*MB [re] [an adult: medical treatment]* [1997]). In this chapter we consider the law relating to mentally incapacitated adults.

The mentally incapacitated adult

Prior to the coming into force of the Mental Capacity Act 2005, the common law position was that health professionals had to act in the best interests of a mentally incapacitated person (*F [re] v West Berkshire H A* [1989]) and follow the reasonable standard of care as laid down in the Bolam Test. This principle was laid down by the House of Lords in a case involving the sterilisation of a woman with learning disabilities. The facts are shown in *Box 8.2*.

Box 8.2 Case *Re F (1989)*

A severely mentally impaired woman had formed an attachment with a fellow patient in a hospital for the mentally handicapped. It was clear that she did not have the capacity to understand or cope with a pregnancy and it was considered that it would be advisable if she were sterilised. However since she was over 18, no one had in law the right to give consent on her behalf.

The House of Lords issued the declaration that the woman in this case could be sterilised. In giving the required declaration, however, the court recommended that while most day-to-day activities performed by professionals on behalf of mentally incapacitated adults could take place under the doctrine of necessity, it wished applications in relation to sterilisations to come before the courts and a Practice Direction covering this was subsequently published.

Mental Capacity Act 2005

The gap in statutory provision relating to decision making on behalf of the mentally incapacitated adult was filled by the Mental Capacity Act 2005. It followed a long period of consultation and debate and most of its provisions came into force in October 2007. It set out statutory principles that should be followed when decisions are made concerning mental capacity. These are shown in *Box 8.3*.

Box 8.3 Statutory principles set out in the Mental Capacity Act 2005

1. A person must be assumed to have capacity unless it is established that he lacks capacity.
2. A person is not to be treated as unable to make a decision unless all practicable steps to help him to do so have been taken without success.
3. A person is not to be treated as unable to make a decision merely because he makes an unwise decision.
4. An act done, or decision made, under this Act for or on behalf of a person who lacks capacity must be done, or made, in his best interests.
5. Before the act is done, or the decision is made, regard must be had to whether the purpose for which it is needed can be as effectively achieved in a way that is less restrictive of the person's rights and freedom of action.

The Mental Capacity Act 2005 also set out a statutory definition of mental capacity which is discussed in *Chapter 6*.

Best interests

Principle 4 (see *Box 8.3*) states that where an act is done or decision is made on behalf of a person who lacks capacity, then it must be done in that person's best interests. The Act does not define 'best interests' but it does set out the steps that should be taken when making such a decision. These are shown in *Box 8.4*.

Box 8.4 Mental Capacity Act 2005 Section 4: Best interests

(1) In determining for the purposes of this Act what is in a person's best interests, the person making the determination must not make it merely on the basis of

    (a) the person's age or appearance, or

    (b) a condition of his, or an aspect of his behaviour, which might lead others to make unjustified assumptions about what might be in his best interests.

(2) The person making the determination must consider all the relevant circumstances and, in particular, take the following steps.

(3) He must consider

    (a) whether it is likely that the person will at some time have capacity in relation to the matter in question, and

    (b) if it appears likely that he will, when that is likely to be.

(4) He must, so far as reasonably practicable, permit and encourage the person to participate, or to improve his ability to participate, as fully as possible in any act done for him and any decision affecting him.

(5) Where the determination relates to life-sustaining treatment he must not, in considering whether the treatment is in the best interests of the person concerned, be motivated by a desire to bring about his death.

(6) He must consider, so far as is reasonably ascertainable

    (a) the person's past and present wishes and feelings (and, in particular, any relevant written statement made by him when he had capacity),

    (b) the beliefs and values that would be likely to influence his decision if he had capacity, and

    (c) the other factors that he would be likely to consider if he were able to do so.

(7) He must take into account, if it is practicable and appropriate to consult them, the views of

    (a) anyone named by the person as someone to be consulted on the matter in question or on matters of that kind,

    (b) anyone engaged in caring for the person or interested in his welfare,

    (c) any donee of a lasting power of attorney granted by the person, and

    (d) any deputy appointed for the person by the court as to what would be in the person's best interests and, in particular, as to the matters mentioned in subsection (6).

(8) The duties imposed by subsections (1) to (7) also apply in relation to the exercise of any powers which

    (a) are exercisable under a lasting power of attorney, or

    (b) are exercisable by a person under this Act where he reasonably believes that another person lacks capacity.

Box 8.4 cont/

Box 8.4/cont

(9) In the case of an act done, or a decision made, by a person other than the court, there is sufficient compliance with this section if (having complied with the requirements of subsections (1) to (7)) he reasonably believes that what he does or decides is in the best interests of the person concerned.

(10) 'Life-sustaining treatment' means treatment which in the view of a person providing health care for the person concerned is necessary to sustain life.

(11) 'Relevant circumstances' are those

    (a) of which the person making the determination is aware, and

    (b) which it would be reasonable to regard as relevant.

Deciding what are a mentally incapacitated person's best interests involves a knowledge of that person's personal views and beliefs, consultation with specified persons and an absence of superficial assumptions based upon appearance, etc.

The case of *Re Y*

In a case (*Y [adult patient] [transplant: bone marrow]* [1996]) heard before the Mental Capacity Act came into force, a judge had to decide whether a bone marrow transplant was in the best interests of a person unable to make her own decisions. A sister suffering from leukaemia wished to check her elder sister's (referred to here as Y) compatibility with her prior to the latter providing a bone marrow transplant. Y suffered both severe physical and mental disabilities and was incapable of giving a valid consent to the blood test or transplant. The court was asked to make a declaration that the blood test and bone marrow could be taken. The court had to decide if this would be in the best interests of Y not the best interests of the younger sister.

The judge argued as follows:

If the sister did not have the bone marrow transplant she would die. This would be a devastating blow to her mother, who suffered from ill health. They were a very close family. The mother would find it more difficult to visit Y in the community home, especially as, after the death of Y's sister, she would then have to look after her only grandchild. Y would suffer as a result of the lack of contact with her mother. The risk of harm to Y from the blood tests was negligible. Although a general anaesthetic posed some risk, it was a low risk. She had already had a general anaesthetic for a hysterectomy without any apparent adverse ill effects. The bone marrow would regenerate. It was to

Y's emotional, psychological and social benefit for her to be a donor. It would therefore be in the best interests of Y for her to have the blood tests and be a donor for her sister.

The declaration that a blood test and, if appropriate, bone marrow harvesting could be taken was therefore issued.

Restraint

It is permissible to use restraint in caring for a mentally incapacitated person provided that the conditions of the Mental Capacity Act 2005 are followed. The use of restraint is defined as including both the decision maker using or threatening to use force to secure the doing of an act which the client/patient resists and also restricts the client/patient's liberty of movement, whether or not he or she resists. The conditions required to make such restraint lawful are:

- that the decision maker must reasonably believe that it is necessary to do the act in order to prevent harm to the client/patient, and
- that the action is a proportionate response.

Proportionate means that the act of restraint is proportionate to both the likelihood of harm to the client/patient and the seriousness of the harm.

Bournewood case and the deprivation of liberty safeguards

The sections in the Mental Capacity Act relating to restraint were amended by the Mental Health Act 2007 so that any restriction of liberty, other than that under the Mental Health legislation must comply with deprivation of liberty safeguards. These safeguards are required as a result of the ruling of the European Court of Human Rights in the Bournewood case that there was a breach of Article 5 of the European Charter on Human Rights when common law powers were used to detain a person lacking mental capacity in a psychiatric hospital (*HL v United Kingdom* [2004]). The amendments to the Mental Capacity Act 2005 by the Mental Health Act 2007 enable a person, over 18 years, suffering from mental disorder and lacking mental capacity to give consent, to be deprived of liberty within the meaning of Article 5, if

- it is in the best interests of the person that he or she be detained as a resident of the hospital or care home in circumstances which amount to a deprivation of liberty; and

- it is necessary that the person be a patient in the hospital or care home in order to prevent harm to him or her,
- it is a proportionate response to the likelihood of suffering harm and the seriousness of that harm.

Six assessments must be carried out:

- Age: The person must be over 18 years.
- Mental health: The person must be suffering from mental disorder as defined by the Mental Health Act as assessed by a doctor.
- Mental capacity: The person must lack the requisite mental capacity as defined in the Mental Capacity Act.
- Best interests: If a deprivation of liberty is occurring, or is going to occur, there must be an assessment as to whether it is in the best interests of the person to be deprived of liberty, whether it is necessary for the person to be so deprived in order to prevent harm to him or herself, and also whether the detention is a proportionate response to the likelihood of the person suffering harm and the seriousness of that harm. The best interests assessor will take into account the views of friends, family members, informal carers and professionals involved in the person's care. If the person is unbefriended, an Independent Mental Capacity Advocate (IMCA) will be appointed to support and represent that person during assessment
- Eligibility: It must be confirmed that the person is not detained under the Mental Health Act 1983 or subject to a conflicting requirement under that Act (e.g. guardianship). If the proposed authorisation relates to deprivation of liberty in a hospital for the purpose of treatment of mental disorder, the assessment will have to establish that there is no evidence that the person objects or would object to mental health treatment. If the person is unable to state any objection, his or her behaviour, wishes, feelings, views, beliefs and values (present and past) should be taken into account.
- Objections: There is no conflict between the authorisation sought and a valid decision by a donee of a lasting power of attorney or a deputy and does not conflict with a valid and applicable advance decision made by the client/patient.

Once these assessments have been carried out, the managers of the hospital or care home can seek authorisation from the primary care trust (in relation to applications from hospitals) or the local authority (in respect of care homes) to deprive the person of liberty for up to one year.

Code of Practice

The Department of Constitutional Affairs prepared a Code of Practice (2007) on the Mental Capacity Act which provides guidance on the Act. This was supplemented by further guidance on the deprivation of liberty safeguards. Both documents can be downloaded from the website (www.justice.gov.uk) of the Ministry of Justice (which replaced the Department of Constitutional Affairs).

Application of the law to the situation in *Box 8.1*

The fact that Julie is occasionally mentally capacitated may mean that she is able to make decisions about her care and treatment in periods of lucidity. However if this is not possible then action needs to be taken in her best interests to ensure that she is receiving pain relief and other care and treatment. The Mental Capacity Act 2005 applies to the situation, and those making decisions on her behalf must ensure that the statutory steps shown in *Box 8.3* are followed. The result is that any views she had about specific treatments which she is no longer able to express can be taken into account. If she had made an advance decision prior to losing the requisite mental capacity then that could be followed (see *Chapter 9*) Minimum restraint, as permitted under the Mental Capacity Act 2005, could be used in her best interests to ensure that she takes the medication. Alternatively there may be justification for her protection in detaining her under the Mental Health Act 1983 to ensure that she receives treatment for her mental disorder.

Conclusion

The Mental Capacity Act 2005 is a welcome provision in facilitating decision making on behalf of those who lack the capacity to make decisions. As cases come before the Court of Protection further guidance on the Act will, together with the Code of Practice, provide greater understanding of the law and more protection for vulnerable adults.

Questions and exercises

1. How does the Mental Capacity Act apply to your area of practice?
2. How do you think that best interests should be defined in relation to pain management decisions?
3. Do you consider that a mentally incapacitated adult should be given the opportunity of altruistic decisions being made on his or her behalf?

References

Department for Constitutional Affairs (2007) *Code of Practice on Mental Capacity Act.* London: DCA

F (re) v West Berkshire H A 1989 2 All ER 545

HL v United Kingdom [2004] ECHR 720 Application No 45508/99 5 October 2004; TLR 19 October 2004

MB (re) (an adult: medical treatment) [1997] 2 FLR 426

Y (re) (adult patient) (transplant: bone marrow) (1996) 35 BMLR 111; [1996] 4 Med LR 204

CHAPTER 9

Living wills/Advance decisions

Box 9.1 Situation

Jane's mother had died of Huntingdon's disease and when Jane discovered that she too was suffering from the same disease, she drew up, whilst still mentally competent a living will, stating that if she lost her mental capacity she would not wish to receive any active intervention to keep her alive and this instruction also included direct oral nutrition and hydration. Her living will was signed by her and also witnessed. Three years later it was apparent that Jane was losing her mental capacity and Jane's daughter brought the living will to the attention of the medical and nursing staff caring for Jane. What is the legal validity of her advance directions?

Introduction

As we saw in *Chapter 6* the treatment decisions of an adult with mental capacity are binding on health professionals. To ignore the refusal to have treatment by a mentally capacitated adult, even if treatment is necessary to save a person's life, is a trespass to the person. This principle also applies to a decision made in advance by a person who is competent at the time of the decision, which is intended to apply at a future time when that person no longer has the mental competence. Such a declaration is known as an advance decision, advance directive, advance refusal or living will.

Common law validity

The principle that an advance statement of refusal is binding derived initially from the common law (i.e. judge-made or case law). In the case concerning Tony Bland (*Airedale NHS Trust v Bland* [1993]) who was in a persistent vegetative state following the Hillsborough stadium disaster, the House of Lords had to decide whether his artificial feeding could be stopped. During its deliberations it stated that had Tony Bland, when competent, drawn up a living will to cover that situation, then the health professionals would have been bound by it. A person is completely at liberty to decline to undergo treatment, even if the result of his so doing will be that he will die. This refusal can be declared in advance.

Mental Capacity Act 2005

Advance refusals of treatment were placed on a statutory footing in the Mental Capacity Act 2005 in accordance with the recommendations of the Law Commission in its report in 1995. This recommendation had initially been rejected in the Government's proposals for decision making on behalf of mentally incapacitated adults (Lord Chancellor, 1999). The White paper published in 1999 stated that it considered that

> *... in the light of the wide range of views on this complex and sensitive subject (i.e. advance statements) and given the flexibility inherent in developing case law, the Government believes that it would not be appropriate to legislate at the present time and thus fix the statutory position once and for all. In rejecting the need for a statute covering living wills, the Government stated (paragraph 16) for the clarity of lawyers, doctors and patients what it perceives to be the present position in law:*
>
> *The current law and medical practice is as follows. It is a principle of law and medical practice that all adults have the right to consent to or refuse medical treatment. Advance statements are a means for patients to exercise that right by anticipating a time when they may lose the capacity to make or communicate a decision.*

Paragraphs 17 to 20 expand on this statement by making it clear that if the advance statement requests specific treatments this does not legally bind a health professional to act contrary to his or her professional judgment. Advance statements do not permit euthanasia 'which is and will remain illegal'.

Statutory provisions

Sections 24 to 26 of the Mental Capacity Act 2005 cover the setting up and validity of an advance decision. Section 24(1) is shown in *Box 9.2*.

The following points are noteworthy:

- A young person under 18 years cannot in law make a binding advance decision. This is because it is possible to overrule a refusal to accept treatment if a person is under 18 years (see *Chapter 7*). However, if a young person under 18 years has drawn up a document setting out his or her views on treatment, that would be taken into consideration in determining what was in his or her best interests (see *Chapter 6*)
- The advance decision only relates to a refusal to have treatment. It

---

Box 9.2 Definition of an advance decision Section 24(1) Mental Capacity Act 2005

Advance decision means a decision made by a person ("P"), after he has reached 18 and when he has capacity to do so, that if

(a) at a later time and in such circumstances as he may specify, a specified treatment is proposed to be carried out or continued by a person providing health care for him, and

(b) at that time he lacks capacity to consent to the carrying out or continuation of the treatment, the specified treatment is not to be carried out or continued.

---

cannot operate as a demand that health professionals provide treatment specified in the document. No professionals can be compelled to carry out treatment that they do not consider to be in the best interests of the patient as the case brought by Burke against the General Medical Council illustrates (*R [on the application of Burke] v General Medical Council and Disability Rights Commission and the Official Solicitor to the Supreme Court* [2004]).

- The person drawing up the advance decision must have the requisite mental capacity at the time his or her wishes are documented. Capacity would be defined in accordance with the Mental Capacity Act (see *Chapter 6*).
- The person must lack the requisite mental capacity at the time the advance decision becomes operative. As long as the maker of the advance decision has the requisite mental capacity, the document has no effect.
- A valid and relevant advance decision must be followed by health professionals.

Format of an advance decision

No specific requirements are laid down for the construction of an advance decision unless it constitutes a refusal of life-sustaining treatment (see below). The Act specifically states that 'a decision may be regarded as specifying a treatment or circumstances even though expressed in layman's terms'.

Withdrawal or alteration of an advance decision

P may withdraw or alter an advance decision at any time when he has capacity to do so and a withdrawal (including a partial withdrawal) need not be in writing. Nor need an alteration be made in writing unless, as a result of the alteration, it comes within the provisions of a refusal relating to life-sustaining treatment.

Refusal of life-sustaining treatment

An advance decision is not applicable to life-sustaining treatment unless

- the decision is verified by a statement by P to the effect that it is to apply to that treatment even if life is at risk, and
- the decision and statement comply with subsection (6).

Subsection 6 requires a refusal relating to life-sustaining treatment to be

- in writing,
- signed by P or by another person in P's presence and by P's direction,
- the signature is made or acknowledged by P in the presence of a witness, and
- the witness signs it, or acknowledges his signature, in P's presence.

Failure to comply with these requirements means that the advance decision will not be effective in its own right of preventing life-sustaining treatment being given, but it may have evidential value in determining what are in the best interests of P.

Validity and relevance of an advance decision

An advance decision is not valid if P

- has withdrawn the decision at a time when he had capacity to do so, or
- has, under a lasting power of attorney, created after the advance decision was made, conferred authority on the donee (or, if more than one, any of them) to give or refuse consent to the treatment to which the advance decision relates*, or
- has done anything else clearly inconsistent with the advance decision remaining his fixed decision.

Nor is an advance decision valid and applicable to the treatment in question if at the material time P has capacity to give or refuse consent to it.
An advance decision is not applicable to the treatment in question if

- that treatment is not the treatment specified in the advance decision,

---

However if there exists a lasting power of attorney which does not give power to the donee to give or refuse consent to treatment to which the advance decision relates then this does not prevent the advance decision from being regarded as valid and applicable.

- any circumstances specified in the advance decision are absent, or
- there are reasonable grounds for believing that circumstances exist which P did not anticipate at the time of the advance decision and which would have affected his decision had he anticipated them.

Effect of an advance decision

If P has made an advance decision which is valid, and applicable to a treatment, the decision has effect as if he had made it, and had had capacity to make it, at the time when the question arises whether the treatment should be carried out or continued. A person does not incur liability for carrying out or continuing the treatment unless, at the time, he is satisfied that an advance decision exists which is valid and applicable to the treatment. A person does not incur liability for the consequences of withholding or withdrawing a treatment from P if, at the time, he reasonably believes that an advance decision exists which is valid and applicable to the treatment.

Concerns over the validity and applicability of an advance decision

Any uncertainty about the validity and applicability of an advance decision can be brought before the Court of Protection which may make a declaration as to whether or not an advance decision exists, is valid, and is applicable to a treatment.

Whilst the validity and applicability of the advance decision is being determined, a person may provide life-sustaining treatment, or do any act he reasonably believes to be necessary to prevent a serious deterioration in P's condition.

Code of Practice Guidance

Guidance has been provided in the Code of Practice on the Mental Capacity Act (Department of Constitutional Affairs, 2007) which can be downloaded from the Ministry of Justice website (www.justice.gov.uk). Chapter 9 of the Code of Practice provides guidance on advance decisions. It is binding on health and social services professionals; attorneys, under a lasting power of attorney; deputies appointed by the Court of Protection; and it is anticipated that informal carers will also find its guidance of value and follow it.

Applying the law to the situation in *Box 9.1*

The provisions of the Mental Capacity Act 2005 apply to Jane's situation. As long as she has the requisite mental capacity to make her own decisions about her treatment, any refusal by her must be respected. She has drawn up a living will and in it she makes an advance refusal of food and hydration. This will only come into effect if she lacks the requisite mental capacity and refers to the treatment which is now under consideration. One difficulty here is that the advance decision only covers treatment and the Code of Practice suggests that since food and hydration is not treatment but basic care, then it cannot be refused in advance by way of an advance decision. There is a lack of clarity in the law here. The Law Commission recommended that it should not be legally possible for a living will to cover basic nursing care. It defined basic nursing care as including pain relief and direct oral nutrition and hydration. Unfortunately this proposal was not specifically included in the Mental Capacity Act 2005 and there are likely to be cases heard before the Court of Protection on what can be refused by means of an advance decision. Following the guidance in the Code of Practice, health professionals would be justified in interpreting Jane's living will as not including oral nutrition and hydration and in continuing to provide that for her. The absence however of statutory provision leaves an uncertainty and until there is a court ruling on the issue, health professionals are in a dilemma as to whether they can lawfully withhold food and drink from Jane on the basis of her living will, or continue to insist that she has direct oral nutrition and hydration contrary to its wording.

Even if the law on advance decisions was interpreted as enabling a person to refuse food and drink at a later time, Jane's advance decision must comply with the requirements relating to a refusal of life-sustaining treatment. Jane has signed the document and it has been witnessed, but she is required to make it clear that she intends to refuse life-sustaining treatment. The absence of such a declaration may mean that her advance directive is not valid and applicable to those treatments. In the event of her advance decision being invalid, her document would stand as an expression of her wishes which could be taken into account in determining what are her best interests (see *Chapter 6*).

Resolving the uncertainty

Faced with these dilemmas, health professionals would be wise to seek the declaration of the court on the validity of the will and its reference to oral nutrition and hydration. Whilst waiting for a decision from the Court of Protection action can be taken to keep Jane alive.

The High Court in the case of *B (re) (consent to treatment: capacity)* had to decide if a mentally capacitated woman was able to ask for her ventilator to be switched off. The decision was that a mentally capacitated adult has the right in law to refuse even life-saving treatment and it was a trespass to her person to treat her without her consent. (See *Chapter 11* for further discussion of this case.)

Conclusions

Statutory provision covering advance decisions is welcome in replacing the common law and making it clear what is the effect of advance refusals and what are the formalities in relation to a refusal of life-sustaining treatment. Some uncertainties still remain in relation to what can be refused and it is hoped that such questions will be resolved in the near future by the Court of Protection.

Questions and exercises

1. What arguments are there in favour of drawing up a living will or advance decision?
2. Do you consider that health professionals should have any discretion in whether or not the directions in a living will should be followed (e.g. in respect of refusal of pain relief or basic nursing care)?
3. What essential features do you consider should be required for a living will to be legally valid?

References

Airedale NHS Trust v Bland [1993] AC 789

B (re) (consent to treatment: capacity) TLR 26 March 2002

British Medical Association (1995) *Advance statements about medical treatment*. London: BMA

Department of Constitutional Affairs (2007) *Code of Practice Mental Capacity Act 2005*. London: Department of Constitutional Affairs

Dimond B (2000) The legal aspects of living wills: A need for clarity. *International Journal of Palliative Care* **6**(6): 304–7

Law Commission (1995) *Mental Incapacity Report No 231*. London: Stationery Office

Lord Chancellor (1999) *Making decisions. The Government's proposals for decision making on behalf of the mentally incapacitated adult*. London: Stationery Office

R (on the application of Burke) v General Medical Council and Disability Rights Commission and the Official Solicitor to the Supreme Court [2004] EWHC 1879; [2004] Lloyd's Rep Med 451

CHAPTER 10

Giving information

Box 10.1 Situation

Mohammad was suffering from severe back pain and sought the advice of an orthopaedic surgeon who advised him that surgery was required to remove a disc which was causing the intractable pain. He was not told that there was a risk of paralysis of the leg if he had this operation. He agreed to the operation and then found that he could not move his left leg. He wishes to sue the surgeon but has been told that the operation was carried out reasonably and there was no negligence in how it was performed. What is his legal situation?

Introduction

In *Chapter 6* it was explained that there were two aspects to the law on consent: the law of trespass and the law of negligence which included the duty of care to inform the patient of significant risks of substantial harm. The law of trespass was considered in *Chapter 6*. This chapter looks at the duty of care in giving information to patients.

The duty of care to inform

The law of negligence is considered in *Chapter 4* where it is pointed out that a duty of care is owed to the patient. The duty of care includes not only a duty to treat and to diagnose it also includes a duty to inform the patient of significant risks of substantial harm. Once a patient has given a valid consent to an operation proceeding, that consent would prevent an action for trespass to the person succeeding. However if the patient has not been given information about the operation which would normally have been given by a health professional following the reasonable standard of care, then an action for negligence may succeed.

The claimant would have to prove on a balance of probabilities the following elements:

- A duty of care was owed to her to inform her of any significant risks of substantial harm.
- There had been a breach of this duty in that the health professional

had not given to her the information that any competent professional following the Bolam Test would have done.

- As a consequence of this failure she agreed to have the operation, which she would not have done had that information been given to her, and
- She has therefore suffered the harm of which she had not been warned.

Sidaway case

The leading case on the giving of information to a patient is that of *Sidaway v Bethlem Royal Hospital Governors* [1985]. The facts are shown in *Box 10.2*.

Box 10.2 The facts of the Sidaway case

The claimant suffered chronic and intractable pain following an operation for a hernia repair. She was eventually referred to a specialist in pain relief who warned her of the possibility of disturbing a nerve root and the possible consequences of so doing but did not mention the possibility of damage to the spinal cord. The risk of spinal cord damage was less than 1%. She consented to the operation which was carried out by the surgeon with due care and skill. However in the course of the operation she suffered injury to her spinal cord which resulted in her being severely disabled. She sued the surgeon for breach of his duty of care to warn her of all possible risks inherent in the operation.

The different judges in the House of Lords all had different bases for their views, but they agreed that in general she had failed in her action. Lord Diplock applied the Bolam principle to the duty of care to inform, Lord Bridge distinguished between two extremes: warning the patient of all possible risks once the treatment has been decided upon in the patient's best interests, not warning the patient of any risks, in order not to alarm the patient. Between these two extremes, Lord Bridge suggested that the Bolam Test should be applied, but this did not mean handing over to the medical profession the entire question of the scope of the duty of disclosure. There will be circumstances where the judge could come to the conclusion that disclosure of a particular risk was so obviously necessary to an informed choice on the part of the patient that no reasonably prudent medical man would fail to make it. Lord Templeman stated that:

In my opinion if a patient knows that a major operation may entail serious consequences, the patient cannot complain of lack of information unless the patient asks in vain for more information or unless there is some danger which by its nature or magnitude or for some other reason required to be separately taken into account by the patient in order to reach a balanced judgment in deciding whether or not to submit to the operation.

Lord Scarman supported a 'prudent patient test', a concept derived from an American case, *Canterbury v Spence*. In this case it was recognised that there were four principles:

1. Every human being of adult years and of sound mind has a right to determine what shall be done with his own body.
2. The consent is the informed exercise of a choice and that entails an opportunity to evaluate knowledgeably the options available and the risks attendant on each.
3. The doctor must therefore disclose all 'material risks'; what risks are 'material' is determined by the 'prudent patient test', which is as follows:
    A risk is … material when a reasonable person, in what the physician knows or should know to be the patient's position, would be likely to attach significance to the risk or cluster of risks in deciding whether or not to forgo the proposed therapy.
4. The doctor has however a therapeutic privilege. This exception is that a reasonable medical assessment of the patient would have indicated to the doctor that disclosure would have posed a serious threat of psychological detriment to the patient.

The House of Lords accepted that English law did not recognise the doctrine of informed consent. Risks should be disclosed to enable the patient to make a rational choice whether to undergo the particular treatment recommended by a doctor. This duty was subject to the doctor's overriding duty to have regard to the best interests of the patient. Accordingly it was for the doctor to decide what information should be given to the patient and the terms in which that information should be couched. The claimant therefore lost her appeal.

It is not easy for patients to establish that had they known of something that they were not told about, they would have refused a particular course of action. There needs to be some causal link between the failure to be given some information and the subsequent conduct of the person concerned. In the following case, the House of Lords reduced the burden on the claimant: it is sufficient, if they can show that they would have made further inquiries or delayed making a decision had they been given the relevant information.

Case: Chester v Afshar

The patient suffered from severe back pain and gave consent to an operation for the removal of three intra-vertebral discs. The patient claimed that the neurosurgeon failed to give a warning to her about the slight risk of post-operative paralysis which the patient suffered following the operation. The trial judge held that the doctor was not negligent in his conduct of the operation, but was negligent in failing to warn her of the slight risk of paralysis which she suffered, and gave judgment for damages to be assessed. The defendant appealed to the Court of Appeal against this finding of failing to give the appropriate information to the claimant.

The Court of Appeal held that the purpose of the rule requiring doctors to give appropriate information to their patients was to enable the patient to exercise her right to choose whether or not to have the particular operation to which she was asked to give her consent. The patient had the right to choose what would and would not be done with her body and the doctor should take the care expected of a reasonable doctor in the circumstances in giving her the information relevant to that choice. The law was designed to require doctors properly to inform their patients of the risk attendant on their treatment and to answer questions put to them as to that treatment and its dangers, such answers to be judged in the context of good professional practice, which had tended to a greater degree of frankness over the years, with more respect being given to patient autonomy.

The object was to enable the patient to decide whether or not to run the risks of having that operation at that time. If the doctor's failure to take care resulted in her consenting to an operation to which she would not otherwise have given her consent, the purpose of that rule would be thwarted if he were not to be held responsible when the very risk about which he failed to warn her materialised and caused her an injury.

The outcome in the Court of Appeal therefore was that the appeal by the surgeon against the finding of negligence in not giving information failed and the patient won the case.

The defendant then appealed to the House of Lords which, by a majority verdict, dismissed the appeal. The House of Lords held that the claimant had shown that had she been notified of the risk of paralysis, which in fact occurred, she would have had to think further about undergoing the surgery and therefore she had established a causal link between the breach and the injury she had sustained and the defendant was liable in damages.

The case of *Chester v Afshar* was followed in a High Court case where Mrs Birch had suffered harm following a catheter angiography, which it was held had been performed without negligence. The amount of compensation had been agreed as £621 000 but liability was disputed. However she obtained compensation since the surgeon failed to discuss with her the imaging methods and their comparative risks and was therefore in breach of the duty of care to inform. The judge held that there was a duty to inform Mrs Birch about comparative risk of the catheter angiography alongside magnetic resonance imaging (MRI). There was no dispute that that duty was breached since the defendant conceded that comparative risks were not raised. The judge stated that

> It is clear to me that had she been given a fair and balanced account in the way I have held was necessary she would have rejected catheter angiography

in favour of MRI. In other words, properly informed she would have declined the procedure leading to her stroke.

(*Birch v University College London Hospital NHS Foundation Trust* [2008])

Application of the law to Mohammad's situation

Mohammad signed the consent form knowing that an operation was to be carried out on his disc. He could not therefore succeed in an action for trespass to the person. Nor is it likely that he could succeed in an action for negligence for failures in the skill and care used in the operation, since he has no evidence that there were such failures. He may however succeed in an action for negligence alleging that there has been a breach of the duty of care to inform him of the significant risks of substantial harm which could occur from the disc operation. He would have to prove on a balance of probabilities that his surgeon failed to give him the information which any competent surgeon following the Bolam Test would have given. In addition he would have to show that had he had that information and knew of the risk of harm, he would have either refused to have had the operation or would have had to think further about undergoing the surgery.

Conclusion

The Kennedy Report (2001) of paediatric heart surgery at Bristol Royal Infirmary emphasised that consent to treatment should be seen as a process and not simply the signing of a form. Feedback from patients should be encouraged. There should be a duty of candour, to tell a patient if adverse events have occurred and patients should receive an acknowledgement, an explanation and an apology. The implementation of such recommendations may move the legal position from the Bolam Test of giving information to the 'prudent patient test' advocated by Lord Scarman in the Sidaway case.

Questions and exercises

1. In what circumstances do you consider that information should be withheld from the patient?
2. Do you follow any specific check-list or principles when giving information to a patient about proposed treatment?
3. Do you encourage patients to read the manufacturer's warnings about the medicines which you prescribe or administer?

References

Birch v University College London Hospital NHS Foundation Trust [2008] EWHC 2237 (QB) (29 September 2008)

Canterbury v Spence 464 F 2d 772 (DC,1972)

Chester v Afshar [2002] TLR, 13 June 2002; 3 All ER 552, CA

Kennedy Report (2001) *Learning from Bristol: The report of the public inquiry into children's heart surgery at the Bristol Royal Infirmary 1984–1995* Command Paper CM 5207. Available from: http://www.bristol-inquiry. org.uk/

Sidaway v Bethlem Royal Hospital Governors and others [1985] 1 All ER 643

CHAPTER 11

Letting die, killing and suicide

> **Box 11.1 Case of *In re B***
>
> Miss B suffered a ruptured blood vessel in her neck which damaged her spinal cord. As a consequence she was paralysed from the neck down and was on a ventilator. She was of sound mind and knew that there was no cure for her condition. She asked for the ventilator to be switched off. Her doctors wished her to try out some special rehabilitation to improve the standard of her care and felt that an intensive care ward was not a suitable location for such a decision to be made. They were reluctant to perform such an action as switching off the ventilator without the court's approval. Ms B applied to court for a declaration to be made that the ventilator could be switched off.

Introduction

In *Chapter 2* we considered the case of Diane Pretty who wanted her husband to be allowed to help her die. In this chapter we consider the law relating to murder and manslaughter and the legal distinction between letting die, killing, suicide and the right of autonomy of the mentally competent adult.

Murder and manslaughter

Murder

In order to secure a conviction of murder, the prosecution has to prove beyond all reasonable doubt that the defendant must either have intended to cause death or intended to cause grievous bodily harm. Unless a situation comparable to that of Dr Shipman, who was convicted of murdering 15 patients, exists, it would be very unusual to be able to prove the intent necessary to convict of murder in a case involving professional care. Following a conviction for murder, a judge at the present time has no discretion over sentencing but must sentence the convicted person to life imprisonment, i.e. a life sentence is mandatory.

Involuntary manslaughter

This may arise where death results from the gross negligence of a health professional where there is no intention to kill or to cause grievous harm. In such cases there may be a prosecution for involuntary manslaughter or there may be no prosecution at all. It depends upon the circumstances. If for example there is such gross negligence leading to the death, then there may be a prosecution for manslaughter. The following two cases illustrate two different situations.

Death by misadventure

In 1991 two junior doctors were given a nine-month suspended prison sentence for the manslaughter of a 16-year-old boy with leukaemia. He died after being wrongly injected in the spine with a cytotoxic drug which should have been administered intravenously. The conviction for manslaughter was quashed by the Court of Appeal on the ground that the jury should have been directed by the judge to decide whether the defendants were guilty of 'gross negligence' and not 'recklessness' and whether there were any mitigating circumstances such as the lack of supervision from more experienced staff (*R v Prentice; R v Adomako; R v Holloway* [1993]).

Manslaughter

In the second case, Dr Adomako, the person charged, was, during the latter part of an operation, the anaesthetist in charge of the patient. At approximately 11.05 a.m. a disconnection occurred at the endotracheal tube connection. The supply of oxygen to the patient ceased and led to a cardiac arrest at 11.14 a.m. During that period the defendant failed to notice or remedy the disconnection. He first became aware that something was amiss when an alarm sounded on the Dinamap machine, which monitored the patient's blood pressure. From the evidence it appeared that some four and a half minutes would have elapsed between the disconnection and the sounding of the alarm. When the alarm sounded the defendant responded in various ways by checking the equipment and by administering atropine to raise the patient's pulse. However, at no stage before the cardiac arrest did he check the integrity of the endotracheal tube connection. The disconnection was not discovered until after resuscitation measures had been commenced.

Dr Adomako accepted at his trial that he had been negligent. The issue was whether his conduct was criminal. He was convicted of involuntary manslaughter but appealed against his conviction. He lost his appeal in the Court of Appeal and then appealed to the House of Lords.

The House of Lords clarified the legal situation. The stages that the House of Lords suggested should be followed were:

1. The ordinary principles of the law of negligence should be applied to ascertain whether or not the defendant had been in breach of a duty of care towards the victim who had died.
2. If such a breach of duty was established the next question was whether that breach of duty caused the death of the victim.
3. If so, the jury had to go on to consider whether that breach of duty should be characterised as gross negligence and therefore as a crime. That would depend on the seriousness of the breach of duty committed by the defendant in all the circumstances in which the defendant was placed when it occurred.
4. The jury would have to consider whether the extent to which the defendant's conduct departed from the proper standard of care incumbent upon him, involving as it must have done a risk of death to the patient, was such that it should be judged criminal.

The judge was required to give the jury a direction on the meaning of gross negligence as had been given in the present case by the Court of Appeal.

The jury might properly find gross negligence on proof of
 1. indifference to an obvious risk of injury to health, or of
 2. actual foresight of the risk coupled either
   (a) with a determination nevertheless to run it or
   (b) with an intention to avoid it but involving such a high degree of negligence in the attempted avoidance as the jury considered justified conviction, or
 3. of inattention or failure to advert to a serious risk going beyond mere inadvertence in respect of an obvious and important matter which the defendant's duty demanded he should address.
                              (Lettering and numbering are the author's)

The House of Lords held that the Court of Appeal had applied the correct test and his appeal was dismissed.

The judge has full discretion over the sentencing in a case of conviction for involuntary manslaughter.

The case of Dr Nigel Cox

Dr Nigel Cox was convicted when he prescribed and administered potassium chloride to a terminally ill patient and was sentenced to a year's imprisonment which was suspended for a year (*R v Cox The Times 22 September 1992*). He also had to appear before disciplinary proceedings of the Regional Health Authority, his employers, and before the General Medical Council.

Voluntary manslaughter

This term is used to cover the situation where the defendant has caused the death of a person with intent but owing to special circumstances a charge or conviction of murder is not appropriate. Prior to the implementation of the Coroners and Justice Act 2009 the term covered:

- death as a result of the provocation of the accused;
- death as a result of diminished responsibility of the accused;
- killing as a result of a suicide pact.

Coroners and Justice Act 2009: Loss of control

Section 56 of the Coroners and Justice Act 2009 abolished the common law defence of provocation to a charge of murder. This is replaced by Section 54 which provides a new partial defence of 'loss of control' to a charge of murder. The effect is to reduce the charge of one of manslaughter if successfully pleaded. The defence of loss of control is shown in *Box 11.2*.

It must be shown that self-control was lost because of a 'qualifying trigger'. The meaning of this is given in Section 55 which is shown in *Box 11.3*.

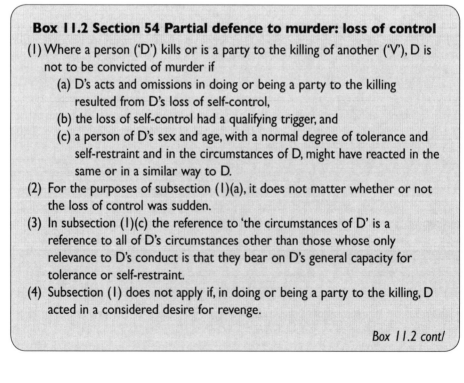

Box 11.2 Section 54 Partial defence to murder: loss of control

(1) Where a person ('D') kills or is a party to the killing of another ('V'), D is not to be convicted of murder if
  (a) D's acts and omissions in doing or being a party to the killing resulted from D's loss of self-control,
  (b) the loss of self-control had a qualifying trigger, and
  (c) a person of D's sex and age, with a normal degree of tolerance and self-restraint and in the circumstances of D, might have reacted in the same or in a similar way to D.
(2) For the purposes of subsection (1)(a), it does not matter whether or not the loss of control was sudden.
(3) In subsection (1)(c) the reference to 'the circumstances of D' is a reference to all of D's circumstances other than those whose only relevance to D's conduct is that they bear on D's general capacity for tolerance or self-restraint.
(4) Subsection (1) does not apply if, in doing or being a party to the killing, D acted in a considered desire for revenge.

Box 11.2 cont/

Box 11.2 Cont/

(5) On a charge of murder, if sufficient evidence is adduced to raise an issue with respect to the defence under subsection (1), the jury must assume that the defence is satisfied unless the prosecution proves beyond reasonable doubt that it is not.

(6) For the purposes of subsection (5), sufficient evidence is adduced to raise an issue with respect to the defence if evidence is adduced on which, in the opinion of the trial judge, a jury, properly directed, could reasonably conclude that the defence might apply.

(7) A person who, but for this section, would be liable to be convicted of murder is liable instead to be convicted of manslaughter.

(8) The fact that one party to a killing is by virtue of this section not liable to be convicted of murder does not affect the question whether the killing amounted to murder in the case of any other party to it.

Box 11.3 Section 55 Meaning of 'qualifying trigger'

(1) This section applies for the purposes of Section 54.

(2) A loss of self-control had a qualifying trigger if subsection (3), (4) or (5) applies.

(3) This subsection applies if D's loss of self-control was attributable to D's fear of serious violence from V against D or another identified person.

(4) This subsection applies if D's loss of self-control was attributable to a thing or things done or said (or both) which
    (a) constituted circumstances of an extremely grave character, and
    (b) caused D to have a justifiable sense of being seriously wronged.

(5) This subsection applies if D's loss of self-control was attributable to a combination of the matters mentioned in subsections (3) and (4).

(6) In determining whether a loss of self-control had a qualifying trigger
    (a) D's fear of serious violence is to be disregarded to the extent that it was caused by a thing which D incited to be done or said for the purpose of providing an excuse to use violence;
    (b) a sense of being seriously wronged by a thing done or said is not justifiable if D incited the thing to be done or said for the purpose of providing an excuse to use violence;
    (c) the fact that a thing done or said constituted sexual infidelity is to be disregarded.

(7) In this section references to 'D' and 'V' are to be construed in accordance with section 54.

Coroners and Justice Act 2009: Diminished responsibility

The Coroners and Justice Act 2009 amends the Homicide Act 1957 to give a new meaning to diminished responsibility. This is shown in *Box 11.4*.

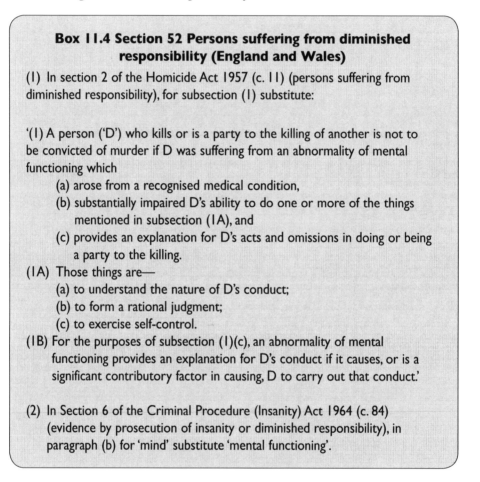

Box 11.4 Section 52 Persons suffering from diminished responsibility (England and Wales)

(1) In section 2 of the Homicide Act 1957 (c. 11) (persons suffering from diminished responsibility), for subsection (1) substitute:

'(1) A person ('D') who kills or is a party to the killing of another is not to be convicted of murder if D was suffering from an abnormality of mental functioning which
    (a) arose from a recognised medical condition,
    (b) substantially impaired D's ability to do one or more of the things mentioned in subsection (1A), and
    (c) provides an explanation for D's acts and omissions in doing or being a party to the killing.
(1A) Those things are—
    (a) to understand the nature of D's conduct;
    (b) to form a rational judgment;
    (c) to exercise self-control.
(1B) For the purposes of subsection (1)(c), an abnormality of mental functioning provides an explanation for D's conduct if it causes, or is a significant contributory factor in causing, D to carry out that conduct.'

(2) In Section 6 of the Criminal Procedure (Insanity) Act 1964 (c. 84) (evidence by prosecution of insanity or diminished responsibility), in paragraph (b) for 'mind' substitute 'mental functioning'.

Letting die: The Tony Bland case (Airedale NHS Trust v Bland [1993])

The House of Lords in the Tony Bland case made it clear that there was in law a clear distinction between letting nature take its course, when, in the light of the prognosis, it was in the best interests not to continue active interventions and killing the patient.

In the word of Lord Goff:

The law draws a crucial distinction between cases in which a doctor decides not to provide, or to continue to provide, for his patient treatment or care which could or might prolong his life and those in which he decides, for example, by administering a lethal drug, actively to bring his patient's life to an end.

The facts of Tony Bland are shown in *Box 11.5*.

Box 11.5 Tony Bland

The patient was a victim of the football stadium crush at Hillsborough and it was established that although he could breathe and digest food independently, he could not see, hear, taste, smell or communicate in any way and it appeared that there was no hope of recovery or improvement. The House of Lords had to decide if it was lawful to permit artificial feeding to be discontinued in the case of a patient in a persistent vegetative state. The House of Lords decided that it would be in the best interests of the patient to discontinue the nasal gastric feed and he was later reported as having died.

A court in Bristol gave consent in a similar case a few months after the House of Lords decision in Tony Bland's case (*Frenchay Healthcare NHS Trust v S* [1994]).

Pain relief and killing

It does not follow that providing appropriate pain relief which may incidentally shorten life is a crime as the trial of Dr Bodkin Adams (*R Adams [Bodkin]* [1957]) made clear. The facts are shown in *Box 11.6*.

Box 11.6 Dr Bodkin Adams

Dr Adams was charged with the murder of a resident of a nursing home in Eastbourne. It was alleged that he gave her large quantities of morphia and heroin which caused her death.

In the case of Dr Bodkin Adams the trial judge Patrick Devlin directed the jury in the following words:

If the first purpose of medicine – the restoration of health – can no longer be achieved, there is still much for the doctor to do, and he is entitled to do all that is proper and necessary to relieve pain and suffering even if the measures he takes may incidentally shorten life ... It remains a fact, and remains a law, that no doctor has the right to cut off life deliberately ... [the defence counsel] was saying that the treatment given by the doctor was designed to promote comfort; and if it was the right and proper treatment of the case, the fact that incidentally it shortened life does not give any grounds for convicting him of murder (Bedford, 1961).

Dr Adams was found not guilty of murder.

Levels of medication

Clearly it must be established that the dosages which are given to a patient in the terminal stages of cancer and other illnesses are in accordance with the reasonable practice of a competent practitioner. It frequently happens that the tolerance built up to some pain medication requires higher and higher doses, which, given to persons without that tolerance would be lethal, grossly negligent and probably amount to a criminal offence. There is considerable benefit when practitioners are treating persons at such high levels to discuss recommended practice with colleagues. The importance of following competent medical practice is shown in the following case.

Annie Lindsell case

On 28 October 1997 Annie Lindsell (Wilkins, 1997) who was terminally ill with motor neurone disease applied to court for a declaration that her GP would not risk prosecution for murder if he gave her potentially lethal painkillers when her condition deteriorated. After hearing that a responsible body of medical opinion supported her GP's plan she withdrew her application for the court's intervention. In the case a clear distinction was made between pain relief whose principal purpose was to control her pain, even though incidentally it might shorten her life, and medication given to end her life. After the hearing, the British Medical Association stated that it was pleased with the outcome

...because it has confirmed that doctors working within the law, can treat the symptoms of terminally ill patients, even if that treatment may have a secondary consequence of shortening the patient's life.

Annie Lindsell died a month later.

Suicide

As a result of the Suicide Act 1969 to attempt to commit suicide ceased to be a crime. However the aiding and abetting of the suicide of another remained a criminal offence under Section 2(1). This is shown in *Box 11.7* as amended by the Coroners and Justice Act 2009.

Box 11.7 Section 2(1) of the Suicide Act 1969 as amended by the Coroners and Justice Act 2009: Section 59 Encouraging or assisting suicide (England and Wales)

(1) The Suicide Act 1961 (c. 60) is amended as follows.

(2) In section 2 (criminal liability for complicity in another's suicide), for subsection (1) substitute:

'(1) A person ('D') commits an offence if

    (a) D does an act capable of encouraging or assisting the suicide or attempted suicide of another person, and

    (b) D's act was intended to encourage or assist suicide or an attempt at suicide.

(1A) The person referred to in subsection (1)(a) need not be a specific person (or class of persons) known to, or identified by, D.

(1B) D may commit an offence under this section whether or not a suicide, or an attempt at suicide, occurs.

(1C) An offence under this section is triable on indictment and a person convicted of such an offence is liable to imprisonment for a term not exceeding 14 years.'

(3) In subsection (2) of that section, for 'it' to the end substitute 'of a person it is proved that the deceased person committed suicide, and the accused committed an offence under subsection (1) in relation to that suicide, the jury may find the accused guilty of the offence under subsection (1).'

(4) After that section insert—

'2A Acts capable of encouraging or assisting

(1) If D arranges for a person ('D2') to do an act that is capable of encouraging or assisting the suicide or attempted suicide of another person and D2 does that act, D is also to be treated for the purposes of this Act as having done it.

(2) Where the facts are such that an act is not capable of encouraging or assisting suicide or attempted suicide, for the purposes of this Act it is to be treated as so capable if the act would have been so capable had the facts been as D believed them to be at the time of the act or had subsequent events happened in the manner D believed they would happen (or both).

(3) A reference in this Act to a person ('P') doing an act that is capable of encouraging the suicide or attempted suicide of another person includes a reference to P doing so by threatening another person or otherwise putting pressure on another person to commit or attempt suicide.

2B Course of conduct

A reference in this Act to an act includes a reference to a course of conduct, and a reference to doing an act is to be read accordingly.'

The effect of the amendments to the Suicide Act 1961 is to bring under the offence of assisting a suicide a person who may not be known to the would-be suicide – such as someone on the Internet – but whose actions encourage the person to attempt to commit suicide.

The opportunity was not taken in Parliament to clarify the law on suicide following the case of Debbie Purdy (see below).

The patient's right of autonomy

In *Chapter 6* we consider the right of autonomy of the mentally capacitated patient and in *Chapter 9* the right of the mentally capacitated patient to refuse, by means of an advance decision, specified treatment if they subsequently lose their mental capacity. In the case of Diane Pretty, which is discussed in *Chapter 2* it is clear that she would have the right to refuse artificial feeding. However she stated that she did not wish to suffer a slow death by starvation and would prefer to have a pain free, dignified and speedy death. In law she could lawfully attempt to commit suicide, but in practice she lacked the physical powers to do so. She therefore needed to have assistance. Her application to the courts for a declaration that her husband should have an immunity from prosecution under Section 2(1) of the Suicide Act 1969 were he to assist her to die, was refused. The House of Lords held that the Suicide Act was not contrary to her human rights as set out in the articles of the European Convention on Human Rights. She then applied unsuccessfully to the European Court of Human Rights in Strasbourg (see *Chapter 2*).

Application of the law to the case in *Box 11.1*

It follows from this that Miss B, whose case is set out in *Box 11.1*, would have been able to refuse to go onto a ventilator. However the anomalous situation which had arisen in her case was that she wished the ventilator to be switched off. She was mentally competent and was able to refuse treatment. However her doctors were reluctant to obey her instructions since it would appear that they would be aiding and abetting a suicide.

The High Court judge held that as a mentally competent adult she had a right to refuse even life-saving treatment. Miss B was awarded a nominal sum of £100 for unlawful trespass. The ventilator could be switched off manually or mechanically and she would be given appropriate palliative drugs to permit her life to end peacefully and with dignity. Other hospitals had said that they would agree to do this. On 29 April 2002 it was announced that Miss B had died peacefully in her sleep after the ventilator had been switched off (*The Times*, 2002).

The President of the Family Division, Dame Elizabeth Butler-Schloss, who heard the case of *B (re) (consent to treatment: capacity)*, restated the principles which had been laid down by the Court of Appeal in the case of St George's Healthcare Trust (*St George's Healthcare NHS Trust v S The Times 8 May 1998* [1999]):

- There was a presumption that a patient had the mental capacity to make decisions whether to consent to or refuse medical or surgical treatment offered.
- If mental capacity was not an issue and the patient, having been given the relevant information and offered the available option, chose to refuse that treatment, that decision had to be respected by the doctors, considerations of what the best interests of the patient would involve were irrelevant.
- Concern or doubts about the patient's mental capacity should be resolved as soon as possible by the doctors within the hospital or other normal medical procedures.
- Meanwhile the patient must be cared for in accordance with the judgment of the doctors as to the patient's best interests.
- It was most important that those considering the issue should not confuse the question of mental capacity with the nature of the decision made by the patient, however grave the consequences. Since the view of the patient might reflect a difference in values rather than an absence of competence the assessment of capacity should be approached with that in mind and doctors should not allow an emotional reaction to, or strong disagreement with, the patient's decision to cloud their judgment in answering the primary question of capacity.
- Where disagreement still existed about competence, it was of the utmost importance that the patient be fully informed, involved and engaged in the process, which could involve obtaining independent outside help, of resolving the disagreement since the patient's involvement could be crucial to a good outcome.
- If the hospital was faced with a dilemma which doctors did not know how to resolve that must be recognised and further steps taken as a matter of priority. Those in charge must not allow a situation of deadlock or drift to occur.
- If there was no disagreement about competence, but the doctors were for any reason unable to carry out the patient's wishes, it was their duty to find other doctors who would do so.
- If all appropriate steps to seek independent assistance from medical experts outside the hospital had failed the hospital should not hesitate to make an application to the High Court or seek the advice of the Official Solicitor.
- The treating clinicians and the hospital should always have in mind that a seriously physically disabled patient who was mentally competent had the same right to personal autonomy and to make decisions as any other person with mental capacity.

Visits to Dignitas

In 2009 the legality of relatives and friends taking a person who wished to end his or her life to the Dignitas clinic in Zurich where a life-ending injection could be given came before the courts. There were over 100 reported cases of people going to Zurich (including a young boy who was not terminally ill but was paralysed) but there had been no prosecutions. Debbie Purdy, who suffered from multiple sclerosis, wanted an assurance that if she delayed her visit to Zurich until such time as she had to rely upon the assistance of her husband, he would not be prosecuted.

Case of Debbie Purdy

Debbie Purdy wished her husband to take her to a Belgian clinic or Switzerland to commit suicide if her condition became unbearably painful and wanted to ensure that he would not be prosecuted for aiding and abetting her suicide (*R [On the application of Purdy] v DPP* [2008]). The High Court dismissed her application that the Director of Public Prosecutions should provide further guidance as to when a prosecution for assisted suicide would be brought. The High Court held that it had great sympathy for Ms Purdy, her husband and others in a similar position to know in advance whether they will face prosecution for doing what many would regard as something that the law should permit, namely to help loved ones to go abroad to end their suffering when they are unable to do it on their own. However it said that this would involve a change in the law. The offence of suicide is very widely drawn to cover all manner of different circumstances: only Parliament can change it. The court also held that the Code of Practice for Crown Prosecutors issued by the Director of Public Prosecutions (DPP), coupled with the general safeguards of administrative law, satisfied human rights convention standards and met the need for clarity and foreseeability and there was no breach of Article 8 of the European Convention on Human Rights and the right to private and family life.

Debbie Purdy was given leave to appeal but the Court of Appeal dismissed her appeal (*R [Purdy] v Director of Public Prosecutions* [February 2009]). It held that she was not entitled to have the specific guidance she was seeking, but that there were broad circumstances in which aiding and abetting suicide would not be prosecuted. Even if there were a prosecution, the court had power to order that the offender should be discharged and might well question publicly the decision to prosecute. It stated that the court was part of the protective system which discouraged and would prevent or extinguish the effect of any arbitrary or unprincipled exercise by the DPP of its responsibilities. The Court of Appeal also said that it was for Parliament to change the law. Ms Purdy said afterwards that she felt that she had won her argument, despite having lost the appeal. She did however appeal to the House of Lords.

The House of Lords, which heard the case on 3 June 2009 gave its judgment on 30 July 2009 (*R [Purdy] v Director of Public Prosecutions* [July 2009]*)*. It unanimously held that the DPP should be required to promulgate a policy identifying the facts and circumstances he would take into account in considering whether to prosecute persons such as the claimant's husband for aiding and abetting an assisted suicide abroad. The lack of clarity on whether there would be a prosecution of relatives who took someone abroad to die was an infringement of Article 8 rights.

Director of Public Prosecution interim policy on assisted suicide prosecutions

On 23 September 2009 the DPP published an interim policy detailing when there would be a prosecution in relation to the offence of assisted suicide. This interim policy set out the following key facts in relation to the DPP's Interim Policy for Prosecutors in respect of Cases of Assisted Suicide:

- Details the public interest factors that Crown Prosecution Service (CPS) prosecutors will consider when deciding whether or not to prosecute someone for assisting suicide (see below).
- Details those public interest factors which carry more weight than others.
- Supplements the Code for Crown Prosecutors, a publicly available document which gives guidance on the general principles to be applied when making decisions about prosecutions.
- Was to apply to all current and future cases until a final policy was published in Spring 2010.
- Applies to all cases where the act(s) of assisting the suicide are carried out in England and Wales, regardless of where the suicide takes place.
- Applies in cases of attempting to assist a suicide.
- Does not address euthanasia which remains murder or manslaughter.
- Does not and cannot provide any individuals with immunity from prosecution.
- Does not and cannot provide an assurance that individuals will be prosecuted.
- Does not and cannot decriminalise assisted suicide.

The full document can be obtained from the Crown Prosecution Service website. The final policy was published in the spring of 2010 following the consultation on the interim policy.

A prosecution is *less likely* to be required if:

- the victim had reached a voluntary, clear, settled and informed decision to commit suicide;
- the suspect was wholly motivated by compassion;

- the actions of the suspect, although sufficient to come within the definition of the offence, were of only minor encouragement or assistance;
- the suspect had sought to dissuade the victim from taking the course of action which resulted in his or her suicide;
- the actions of the suspect may be characterised as reluctant encouragement or assistance in the face of a determined wish on the part of the victim to commit suicide;
- the suspect reported the victim's suicide to the police and fully assisted them in their enquiries into the circumstances of the suicide or the attempt and his or her part in providing encouragement or assistance.

A prosecution is *more likely* to be required if:

- the victim was under 18 years of age;
- the victim did not have the capacity (as defined by the Mental Capacity Act 2005) to reach an informed decision to commit suicide;
- the victim had not reached a voluntary, clear, settled and informed decision to commit suicide;
- the victim had not clearly and unequivocally communicated his or her decision to commit suicide to the suspect;
- the victim did not seek the encouragement or assistance of the suspect personally or on his or her own initiative;
- the suspect was not wholly motivated by compassion; for example, the suspect was motivated by the prospect that he or she or a person closely connected to him or her stood to gain in some way from the death of the victim;
- the suspect pressured the victim to commit suicide;
- the suspect did not take reasonable steps to ensure that any other person had not pressured the victim to commit suicide;
- the suspect had a history of violence or abuse against the victim;
- the victim was physically able to undertake the act that constituted the assistance (to) him or herself;
- the suspect was unknown to the victim and encouraged or assisted the victim to commit or attempt to commit suicide by providing specific information via, for example, a website or publication;
- the suspect gave encouragement or assistance to more than one victim who were not known to each other;
- the suspect was paid by the victim or those close to the victim for his or her encouragement or assistance;
- the suspect was acting in his or her capacity as a medical doctor, nurse, other healthcare professional, a professional carer (whether for payment or not), or as a person in authority, such as a prison officer, and the victim was in his or her care;

- the suspect was aware that the victim intended to commit suicide in a public place where it was reasonable to think that members of the public may be present;
- the suspect was acting in his or her capacity as a person involved in the management or as an employee (whether for payment or not) of an organisation or group, a purpose of which is to provide a physical environment (whether for payment or not) in which to allow another to commit suicide.

The General Medical Council has drafted a consultation document *End of Life Treatment and Care* which was considered at its meeting in February 2010. The finalised guidance can be seen on the GMC website.

As noted above, Parliament failed to take the opportunity to clarify when prosecution for assisted suicide should take place and simply amended the Suicide Act 1961 to extend the offence to cover those who encourage suicide through the Internet or other non-personal ways. Parliament did debate excluding from the criminal offence of assisting a suicide those who accompanied relatives abroad to enable their lives to be ended, but in the end, Parliament ruled against any lightening of the law relating to assisted suicide. Instead it amended the 1961 Act to ensure that those who encouraged others to commit suicide over the Internet could be prosecuted. The amended legislation is shown in *Box 11.7*.

Conclusion

To some philosophers in the ethics of healthcare, the present distinction in law between the legality of letting die (where appropriate) and the illegality of killing is not sustainable in logic, since death is the outcome of both, and killing may cause less suffering that letting nature take its course. The distinction is clearly apparent in a comparison of the cases of Diane Pretty and Miss B. The distinction is however of extreme importance in the law and there is little likelihood of the law being changed in the near future. It remains to be seen if the final guidance issued by the DPP is sufficiently clear for relatives and friends who wish, without fear of prosecution, to support a person to end his or her life when a terminal illness has reached an intolerable situation. If not, Parliament will be compelled to look again at the wording of the Suicide Act 1969.

Questions and exercises

1. Do you consider that a competent adult could refuse every kind of care and treatment?
2. What protection do you consider that the health professional and the patient should have when administering or receiving high dosages of medication?

3. What are the advantages and disadvantages of introducing a law of euthanasia into this country?

References

Airedale NHS Trust v Bland [1993] AC 789

B (re) (consent to treatment: capacity) Report 26 March 2002

Bedford S (1961) *The Best We Can Do*. Harmondsworth: Penguin

Frenchay Healthcare NHS Trust v S [1994] 2 All ER 403

R Adams (Bodkin) [1957] Crim LR 365

R v Adomako House of Lords TLR July 4 1994; [1994] 2 All ER 79

R v Cox The Times 22 September 1992 (1992) 12 BMLR 38

R v Prentice; R v Adomako; R v Holloway [1993] 4 All ER 935

R (On the application of Purdy) v Director of Public Prosecutions [2008] The Times Law Report 17 November 2008

R (Purdy) v Director of Public Prosecutions TLR 24 February 2009

R (Purdy) v Director of Public Prosecutions TLR 31 July 2009 HL

St George's Healthcare NHS Trust v S The Times 8 May 1998 [1999] Fam 26

Wilkins E (1997) Dying woman granted wish for dignified end. *The Times* 29 October

The Times (2002) Miss B dies in peace after treatment ends. *The Times* 30 April

CHAPTER 12

Confidentiality

> **Box 12.1 Situation**
> Jan had multiple sclerosis and in recent weeks had been suffering considerable pain and discomfort and her mobility was becoming increasingly impaired. She told her community nurse that she felt that she could not go on for much longer and was considering taking her own life. She did not ask the nurse for assistance, but requested that the nurse should keep this information confidential. What is the nurse's position in law?

Introduction

There are several sources that give rise to the duty of confidentiality which are recognised by all health professionals. They are explained in the author's book in this healthcare law series (Dimond, 2002). The duty of confidentiality derives from the trust that is created between patient and professional, from the professional codes of practice of registered health professionals and from specific statutory provisions. If there is a breach of confidentiality which is not justified in law, then the patient can apply for an injunction to prevent its publication, if in time, or, if not, sue for damages for the breach of confidentiality. In the case of *X v Y* [1988] doctors working in the NHS who were suffering from AIDS were granted an injunction against a newspaper preventing it publishing their names. The Court held that the information obtained from hospital records should be kept confidential and the public interest did not require the publication of the names. The Court did not order the disclosure by the press of their informant as the circumstances did not constitute one of the exceptional grounds on which the disclosure could be ordered against the press.

Exceptions to the duty of confidentiality

The basic presumption is that confidentiality should be respected but there are specific exceptions recognised both in statute and at common law. These include the following recognised exceptions:

- Consent of the patient.
- Information given to other professionals in the interests of the patient.
- Order from the court before or during legal proceedings.
- Statutory justification, e.g.:
    Notification of registration of births and still births.
    Infectious Disease Regulations.
    Police and Criminal Evidence Act.
- Public interest.

Consent of the patient

When the patient gives consent to the disclosure of confidential information, and the disclosure is made in accordance with this consent, then this would be a complete defence to any allegation of breach of confidentiality. There are clear advantages therefore in obtaining the consent of the patient before disclosure is made, and preferably in writing.

Public interest

Even where the patient refuses to give consent to the disclosure, disclosure may be justified in the public interest. Where harm is feared to the patient or to another person, then the public interest would justify disclosure. For example a concern that a child was at risk of being physically or mentally harmed would require disclosure to the appropriate child protection authorities. Most registration bodies of health practitioners recognise the 'public interest' as being a justification for the disclosure of confidential information. The Court of Appeal in the case of *W v Egdell* [1990] held that an independent psychiatrist who had sent his report to the Home Office and Medical Director of the Hospital was justified in the public interest in making his findings known to those authorities.

Data Protection Act 1998

This Act applies to all patient records, both those that are held in manual format and those held on computer. All such records must comply with the data protection principles and the access provisions set out in statutory instruments (see below). The Information Commissioner combines the roles of Data Protection Commission enforcing the provisions of the Data Protection Act 1998 and Information Commissioner implementing the provisions of the Freedom of Information Act 2000.

The Data Protection Act principles are shown in *Box 12.2*.

Box 12.2 Principles of the Data Protection Act

1. Personal data shall be processed fairly and lawfully and, in particular, shall not be processed unless:
   (a) at least one of the conditions in Schedule 2 is met; and
   (b) in the case of sensitive personal data, at least one of the conditions in Schedule 3 is also met.
2. Personal data shall be obtained only for one or more specified and lawful purposes, and shall not be further processed in any manner incompatible with that purpose or those purposes.
3. Personal data shall be adequate, relevant and not excessive in relation to the purpose or purposes for which they are processed.
4. Personal data shall be accurate and, where necessary, kept up to date.
5. Personal data processed for any purpose or purposes shall not be kept for longer than is necessary for that purpose(s).
6. Personal data shall be processed in accordance with the rights of data subjects under this Act.
7. Appropriate technical and organisational measures shall be taken against unauthorised or unlawful processing of personal data and against accidental loss or destruction of, or damage to, personal data.
8. Personal data shall not be transferred to a country or territory outside the European Economic Area unless that country or territory ensures an adequate level of protection for the rights and freedoms of data subjects in relation to the processing of personal data.

Access to personal health records

Section 7 of the Data Protection Act 1998 enables an individual to be informed of data held about him or her and to access that data. Special provisions exist in relation to health, education and social work under Section 30. Section 30 enables the Secretary of State to draw up specific provisions setting exemptions from the statutory rights of access in relation to health, education and social work records. Statutory Instruments have been enacted setting out details of the restrictions on access to these records (Data Protection [Subject Access Modification] [Health] Order 2000).

Right to withhold access

Access can be withheld under the Data Protection Act 1998 in the following circumstances:

• Where, in the opinion of the holder of the record, serious harm would be caused to the mental or physical health or condition of the applicant or of any other individual.

- Where the identity of a third person would be made known and this person has not consented to access. (This does not apply where the other person is the health professional caring for the patient.)
- Where the reports are confidential under a statutory provision such as information supplied in a report or other evidence given to the court by a local authority, Health or Social Services Board, Health and Social Services Trust or probation officer.

Article 8 of the European Convention on human rights

Article 8 recognises a right to respect for private and family life, home and correspondence and can be invoked where a person is concerned that a public authority or organisation exercising functions of a public nature is breaching or has breached a person's right to confidentiality. The rights bestowed under Article 8 are not absolute, however, and, as can be seen from Appendix 1 paragraph 2, provide qualifications on the right recognised in paragraph 1.

> *There shall be no interference by a public authority with the exercise of this right except such as is in accordance with the law and is necessary in a democratic society in the interests of national security, public safety or the economic wellbeing of the country, for the prevention of disorder or crime, for the protection of health or morals, or for the protection of the rights and freedoms of others.*

There have been many cases where the media have argued that the right to freedom of expression under Article 10 took precedence over an individual's right to privacy under Article 8. For example, Naomi Campbell sued the Mirror Group Newspapers for breach of confidence (*Campbell v MGN Ltd* [2004]). The House of Lords, in a majority decision, held that even though she had brought into the public domain the fact that she was being treated for drug addiction, certain information could still be kept confidential, including the time, form and place of the drug therapy and she was therefore entitled to damages against the Mirror Group Newspapers for that breach of confidence. In this respect her right to privacy succeeded against the right to freedom of expression under Article 10.

Code of Practice on confidentiality

The Department of Health has prepared a Code of Practice on confidentiality which can be accessed on its website (www.dh.gov.uk).

Application of access provisions to a pain management situation

Whilst there is a presumption in favour of access to health records, access could be refused if serious harm was feared. Thus a patient who was terminally ill, but had not at that time been given the diagnosis, could be refused access if there was evidence that serious harm would be caused to his or her physical or mental health or condition. Such an exclusion from access would have to be justified in each case, since the patient has the right to challenge the refusal to provide access. A blanket policy of preventing access is legally invalid.

Application of the law to the situation in *Box 12.1*

Clearly, serious harm is feared to Jan if she continues with her suicide bid. The community nurse has a duty to ensure that Jan is receiving all the palliative care available and that Jan's mental capacity to make her own decisions is assessed. It may be, for example, that Jan needs to receive counselling assistance, since it may be that depression has undermined her mental capacity. She may benefit from further services for mobility and aid from the local authority. The community nurse has to use her professional discretion as to whether it is in Jan's interests for her suicide wishes to be made known to 'others' and who the appropriate 'others' may be. It may be that eventually, the community nurse decides that Jan has all the care that she needs, and that her decision to take her own life is the result of clear thinking by a mentally competent person. If no other person is involved to assist (which would be a criminal offence – see *Chapter 11*) the community nurse may be justified in keeping the disclosure confidential. She may wish to seek advice and guidance from a senior manager or clinical supervisor. It is essential that she keeps clear, comprehensive records of her knowledge and of her actions.

Conclusion

Whether a particular situation justifies a breach of confidentiality in the public interest is ultimately a question of professional discretion. Guidance is provided by the codes of practice and conduct issued by registration bodies, but the application of this guidance to a specific situation has to be decided by the individual practitioner who would be held personally and professionally accountable for his or her decision. Clear and comprehensive documentation is essential.

Questions and exercises

1. In what circumstances would you breach the confidentiality of the patient? What would you tell the patient?

2. Do you consider that there should be an absolute right of access for a patient to his or her health records?
3. The Government is preparing for the introduction of an individual patient electronic record. How would this affect your record keeping practice and what you record?

References

Campbell v MGN Ltd [2004] *UKHL 22,* [2004] 2 A.C. 457 HL

Data Protection (Subject Access Modification)(Health) Order 2000 SI 2000 No 413; Data Protection (Subject Access Modification)(Education) Order 2000 SI 2000 No 414; Data Protection (Subject Access Modification) (Social Work) Order 2000 SI 2000 No 415

Dimond B (2002) *The Legal Aspects of Patient Confidentiality.* Dinton, Wiltshire: Quay Books Mark Allen Publishing

W v Egdell [1990] 1 All ER 835

X v Y [1988] 2 All ER 648

CHAPTER 13

Medicines

Box 13.1 Situation

Augusta is a palliative care nurse who visits patients in the community advising them, their relatives and GPs on their care, and arranging admissions to the hospice when appropriate. One patient is in the terminal stages of renal failure and on high doses of morphine. She is clearly in considerable discomfort and Augusta is asked by the patient if she could increase her dose. The patient does not wish her relatives to be told. Augusta is anxious to do this as soon as possible, since it may be several hours before the GP is able to visit. She phones the GP who tells her that she can give an additional dose and he would write it up later. Augusta administers this additional dose. Before the doctor has written up the additional dose, the patient dies. The relatives are now claiming that Augusta killed the patient. What is the law?

Introduction

The 1968 Medicines Act provided a statutory framework for the supply and control of medicines and sets out the classification of drugs. The Misuse of Drugs Act 1971 and subsequent legislation regulates the supply of specified controlled drugs. These statutes have been supplemented by Statutory Instruments providing more detailed regulation.

Previously, the Medicines Control Agency (MCA) had the function of monitoring the safety and quality of medicines. Its website provided access for health professionals, members of the public, academics, the pharmaceutical industry and journalists. It operated a Defective Medicines Report Centre. However, on 1 April 2003 the Medicines Control Agency merged with the Medical Devices Agency to form the Medicines and Healthcare Products Regulatory Agency (MHRA). The Department of Health considered that this merger would provide the opportunity to build on the undoubted strengths of the MCA and would continue to be a world leader in terms of its scientific expertise.

While initially under the Medicines Act 1968 the only recognised professions for prescribing medications were doctors, dentists, veterinary surgeons and midwives, legislation over the past 17 years has expanded approved prescribers.

Nurse prescribing

Following the first Crown Report (Department of Health, 1989) the powers of prescribing were extended to nurses and health visitors. The Medicinal Products (Nurse Prescribing etc) Act 1992 enables a registered nurse, either health visitor or district nurse, who has the requisite additional training to prescribe those medicinal products contained in a nurse's formulary, set out in a Schedule to the Prescription Only Medicines Order (Statutory Instrument Prescription Only Medicines 1994). Section 58 of the Medicines Act 1968 (as Amended by the 1992 Act) enables an appropriate practitioner to provide a prescription to be dispensed by the registered pharmacist. Nurse prescribing in the community therefore has a clear statutory basis and can take place within certain clearly defined parameters (Dimond, 1995). Further amending regulations relating to nurse prescribing were made in 1997 (Prescription Only Medicines [Human Use] Order 1977 SI 1997/1830).

In February 2000 an amendment by Statutory Instrument added nurses employed by a doctor whose name is included in a medical list (e.g. practice nurses) and those assisting in the capacity of a nurse, in the provision of services in a walk-in centre defined as a centre at which information and treatment for minor conditions is provided to the public under arrangements made by or on behalf of the Secretary of State to the group of nurses who were recognised as being able to prescribe after the appropriate training had been given.

Second Crown Report and patient group directions

Dr Crown was appointed in 1997 to review prescribing, supply and administration of medicines. The terms of reference included the development of a consistent policy framework to guide judgments on the circumstances in which health professionals might undertake new responsibilities with regard to prescribing, supply and administration of medicines. It was also asked to advise on the likely impact of any proposed changes; to consider possible implications for legislation, professional training and standards; and to advise on prescription etc. under group protocols and on any safeguards.

The initial report was published in 1998 and was concerned with the prescribing, supply and administration under group protocols (Department of Health, 1998). It recommended that the majority of patients should continue to receive medicines on an individual basis. However current safe and effective practice using group protocols which are consistent with criteria defined in the Report should continue. As a consequence of this interim Report a statutory instrument was published specifying the minimum requirements for a patient group direction (originally known as group protocol). These requirements are shown in *Box 13.2*.

One developing role of the practitioner specialising in pain management

Box 13.2 Particulars for patient group direction

(a) The period during which the direction shall have effect

(b) The description or class of prescription only medicines to which the direction relates

(c) Whether there are any restrictions on the quantity of medicine which may be supplied on any one occasion, and if so, what restrictions

(d) The clinical situations which prescription only medicines of that description or class may be used to treat

(e) The clinical criteria under which a person shall be eligible for treatment

(f) Whether any class of person is excluded from treatment under the direction, and if so, what class of person

(g) Whether there are circumstances in which further advice should be sought from a doctor or dentist and, is so, what circumstances

(h) The pharmaceutical form or forms in which prescription only medicines of that description or class are to be administered

(i) The strength, or maximum strength, at which prescription only medicines of that description or class are to be administered

(j) The applicable dosage or maximum dosage

(k) The route of administration

(l) The frequency of administration

(m) Any minimum or maximum period of administration applicable to prescription only medicines of that description or class

(n) Whether there are any relevant warnings to note, and if so, what warnings

(o) Whether there is any follow up action to be taken in any circumstances, and if so, what action and in what circumstances

(p) Arrangements for referral for medical advice

(q) Details of the records to be kept of the supply or the administration of medicines under the direction.

is the transcribing of patient group directions on ward drug charts for nurse prescribing. The specialist nurse could, within the agreed patient group direction, amend the drug charts to suit the changing needs of the patient and write up drugs for ward charts to be administered by the ward nurses.

The final Crown Report

The recommendations of the Final Report of the Crown Committee (Department of Health, 1999) included the following recommendations:

1. The legal authority in the UK to prescribe should be extended beyond currently authorised prescribers.

2. The legal authority to prescribe should be limited to medicines in specific therapeutic areas related to particular competence and expertise of the group.
3. Two types of prescribers should be recognised: the independent prescriber and the dependent (now known as the supplementary) prescriber.
4. A UK-wide advisory body, provisionally entitled the 'New Prescribers Advisory Committee' should be established under Section 4 of the Medicines Act to assess submissions from professional organisations seeking powers for suitably trained members to become independent or dependent prescribers.
5. Newly authorised groups of prescribers should not normally be allowed to prescribe specified categories of medicines including controlled drugs.
6. The current arrangements for the administration and self-administration of medicines should continue to apply. Newly authorised prescribers should have the power to administer those parenteral prescription only medicines which they are authorised to prescribe.

As a consequence of these recommendations, legislation was contained in Section 63 of the Health and Social Care Act which amended the Medicines Act 1968. It amended Section 58 of the Medicines Act to enable

...other persons who are of such a description and comply with such conditions as may be specified in the order...

to be eligible to write prescriptions for medicinal products.

Section 63(3) lists those persons who are eligible as including persons who are registered by a board established under the Professions Supplementary to Medicine Act 1960 or by a body set up under the Health Act 1999 (for example the Health Professions Council or the Nursing and Midwifery Council).

Supplementary prescribers

In April 2002 the Department of Health (2002a) announced its intention of introducing supplementary prescribing by a nurse or pharmacist in 2003. The aim was to enable the pharmacists and nurses to work in partnership with doctors and help treat such conditions as asthma, diabetes, high blood pressure and arthritis. The doctor would draw up a plan with the patient's agreement, laying out the range of medicines that may be prescribed and when to refer back to the doctor. Further details of the patient conditions and the medicinal products that would be the subject of supplementary prescribing were given in November 2002 (Department of Health, 2002b). In April 2005 chiropodists and podiatrists, physiotherapists and radiographers were added to list of those who could become supplementary prescribers and restrictions on their prescribing controlled drugs or unlicensed medicines were removed. (The National Health Service [Primary Medical Services] Miscellaneous Amendments Regulations SI 2005). The supplementary prescriber works within a Clinical Management Plan (CMP) agreed with the independent prescriber. The Medicines and Healthcare Regulatory Agency published guidance on supplementary prescribing in 2003.

Extended Formulary nurse prescribers

Further developments in extending prescribing powers came into force on 1 April 2002. The Prescription Only Medicines (Human Use) Amendment Order Statutory Instrument 2002 laid down arrangements for a nurse registered in Parts 1, 3, 5, 8, 10, 11, 12, 13, 14, or 15 of the professional register and who was recorded in the register as qualified to order drugs, medicines and appliances from the Extended Formulary to prescribe products listed in the Extended Formulary. Schedule 3A of the statutory instrument set out the substances which may be prescribed, administered or directed for administration by Extended Formulary nurse prescribers. The Schedule also set out the conditions for such prescription or administration. The list included antibiotics, analgesics and vaccines. Full details were published in the *British National Formulary*. In brief, the Extended Formulary nurse prescribers were able to prescribe all pharmacy and general sales list medicines prescribable by a GP and also those Prescription Only medicines which were set out in Schedule 3A of the Order. These covered minor injuries, minor ailments, health promotion and palliative care.

Guidance on extending independent nurse prescribing within the NHS in England

Guidance was issued in March 2002 by the Department of Health (2002c). It covered such topics as who may prescribe and what; implementation strategy; education and training; action for employers; prescription form; security and handling of prescription forms; good practice; nursing records; adverse reaction reporting; legal and clinical liability; dispensing of prescribed items; verification of prescribing status; dispensing and budget setting and monitoring.

On 16 April 2002 the Department of Health (2002a) published proposals to give nurses and pharmacists further prescribing powers to cover some chronic conditions. The proposals were implemented in 2003 and enable appropriately trained nurses and pharmacists to prescribe for such conditions as asthma, diabetes, high blood pressure and arthritis. Prescriptions for inhalers, hormone replacement therapy and anti-coagulants were also included.

From 1 May 2006 further amendments were made to the prescribing powers of nurses (Statutory Instrument [2006] 1015). District nurse/health visitor formulary nurses and any nurse undertaking a V100 prescribing programme as part of a Specialist Practitioner qualification are known as community practitioner nurse prescribers (V100). Health visitors are now known as specialist community public health nurses. From 2006 the term extended formulary prescriber has been dropped and the term nurse independent prescriber is used. Prescribing by the independent nurse prescriber is not limited to a specified formulary but must of course be within the field of experience, training and knowledge of the nurse.

Standards for medicines management

The Nursing and Midwifery Council (NMC) published in 2008 *Standards for Medicines Management* which sets standards over 10 areas. These include: methods of supplying and/or administration of medicines; dispensing; storage and transportation; standards for practice of administration of medicines; delegation; disposal; unlicensed medicines; complementary and alternative therapies; management of adverse events; and controlled drugs. Standards of good practice are set in each section.

Independent nurse prescribers

In May 2006 the Nurse Prescribers' Extended Formulary was discontinued and qualified nurse independent prescribers are now able to prescribe any licensed medicine for any medical condition within their competence, including some controlled drugs (National Health Service [Miscellaneous Amendments Relating to Independent Prescribing] Regulations 2006). Further information is available from the Department of Health website. A nurse independent prescriber means a person (a) who is a registered nurse or registered midwife and (b) against whom is recorded in the professional register an annotation signifying that he or she is qualified to order drugs, medicines and appliances as a nurse independent prescriber or a nurse independent/supplementary prescriber. Nurse independent prescribers are only able to prescribe or administer a limited range of controlled drugs as set out in Schedule 3A of the Statutory Instrument. Independent prescribing by pharmacists is also facilitated.

The NMC published in 2006 *Standards of Proficiency for Nurse and Midwife Prescribers*. This document has four sections covering education and training provision to prepare nurses and midwives to prescribe, 21 standards for prescribing practice, additional guidance, and further information. The 21 standards for prescribing practice include 'licence as a prescriber', accountability, assessment, need, consent, communication, record keeping, clinical management plans (supplementary prescribing), prescribing and administration/supply, prescribing and dispensing, prescribing for family and others, computer-generated prescribing by nurses or midwives, evidence-based prescribing, delegation, continuing professional development, controlled drugs, prescribing unlicensed medicines, prescribing medicines for use outside the terms of the licence, repeat prescribing, remote prescribing via telephone, email, fax, video link or website, and gifts and benefits.

Controlled drugs

The fourth Shipman Inquiry made radical recommendations on controlled drugs which led to legislative changes in the Health Act 2006. Sections 17 to 25 introduced new laws in relation to the supervision of management, and use of controlled drugs, and regulations strengthened the governance and monitoring arrangements for controlled drugs (The Controlled Drugs [Supervision of Management and Use] Regulations 2006). An Accountable Officer must now be appointed within each trust to have responsibility for the safe use and management of controlled drugs. The guidance builds on the safe and secure handling of medicines (known as the revised Duthie Report, March 2005). In addition, amendments to the Misuse of Drugs Regulations enable all details on prescriptions for controlled drugs except the signature to be computer generated and the computerisation of controlled drugs registers for drugs listed in Schedule 2 and 3. The final changes to record keeping requirements can be obtained from the Department of Health (2006). Powers are given to a constable or other authorised person to enter and inspect premises and stocks and records of controlled drugs. Further information can be found in the joint paper published by the Department of Health and the Royal Pharmaceutical Society of Great Britain on the safer management of controlled drugs (2007).

Application of the law to the situation in *Box 13.1*

Many palliative care practitioners have, after the appropriate training which is financed from central funds, become eligible to be independent nurse prescribers. Further details of the Department of Health guidance is available from its website (www.dh.gov.uk/). The answer to the situation therefore depends upon Augusta's status in relation to prescribing. She may have done the training and be qualified as an independent prescriber. If so, then she would have the power to prescribe the necessary medication for the patient. However, on the facts given here and the fact that the GP has prescribed the medication, it does not appear that Augusta is an independent prescriber. She may have the powers of prescribing as a supplementary prescriber. If so, she may be able to prescribe the additional controlled drugs, depending upon the details of her supplementary prescribing arrangements. The supplementary prescribing regulations require the independent prescriber to be a doctor or a dentist; the registered nurse or midwife to have an annotation in the register that she is qualified to order drugs, medicines and appliances as a supplementary prescriber; that there is a written clinical management plan relating to the named patient and to that patient's specific conditions; that agreement to this clinical management plan is recorded by both the independent and the supplementary prescribers before the plan is implemented; and both independent and supplementary prescriber share access to, consult and use the same common patient record. If all these conditions are met, then Augusta can lawfully amend the patient's prescription in accordance with the plan.

If, however, Augusta is neither an independent nor a supplementary prescriber, she does not have power to change the prescription and the situation is one where she is carrying out instructions given by a doctor over the telephone with all the dangers that ensue. Standard 11 of the NMC Standards of Medicine Management (Nursing and Midwifery Council, 2008) states that:

> In exceptional circumstances, where medication has been previously prescribed and the prescriber is unable to issue a new prescription, but where changes to the dose are considered necessary, the use of information technology (such as fax, text message or email) may be used but must confirm any change to the original prescription.

If Augusta has made changes to the prescription without appropriate authorisation, then she is clearly guilty of misconduct. She should have waited for the doctor to attend the patient. It is however unlikely that her actions caused the death of the patient (although this would have to be investigated). She could face prosecution and disciplinary actions before her employers and also professional conduct proceedings before the NMC.

Conclusions

The extension of independent and supplementary prescribing and the use of patient directions has made a huge impact on the ability to deliver immediate services to patients. There are however dangers that too casual an attitude to prescribing powers could lead to patients being harmed. It is essential that there should be sufficient on-going training and that prescribers should always work within their competence and ensure that they keep up to date on information about the substances they can prescribe. These developments have a major impact upon the role of the palliative care nurse and all those health professionals concerned with pain management.

Questions and exercises

1. To what extent do you consider that your powers to prescribe could be extended or initiated?
2. Do you consider the present provisions for the safety of medicines provide adequate protection for the patient?

3. How much information do you give a patient about the potential side effects of medication? (Refer also to *Chapter 10*.)

References

Controlled Drugs (Supervision of Management and Use) Regulations 2006 SI No 3148

Department of Health (1989) *Report on Nurse Prescribing and Supply, Advisory Group Chaired by Dr June Crown*. London: HMSO

Department of Health (1998) *Statutory Instrument 2000 No 121 The Review of Prescribing, Supply and Administration of Medicines: A Report on the Supply and Administration of Medicines Under Group Protocols*. London: HMSO

Department of Health (1999) *Final Report on the Prescribing, Supply and Administration of Medicines. Chaired by Dr June Crown*. London: HMSO

Department of Health (2002a) *Groundbreaking New Consultation Aims to Extend Prescribing Powers for Pharmacists and Nurses*. Press release 2002/0189

Department of Health (2002b) *Pharmacists to Prescribe for the First Time. Nurses will Prescribe for Chronic Illness*. Press release 2002b/0488

Department of Health (2002c) *Extending Independent Nurse Prescribing Within the NHS in England. A Guide for Implementation*. London: HMSO

Department of Health (2006) *Safer Management of Controlled Drugs. Changes to Record Keeping Requirements*. DH Gateway Ref. 7187. London: Department of Health

Department of Health and Royal Pharmaceutical Society of Great Britain (2007) *Safer Management of Controlled Drugs*. London: HMSO

Dimond BC (1995) *Nurse Prescribing*. London: Merck Dermatology and Scutari Press

Medicines and Healthcare Products Regulatory Agency (2003) *Supplementary Prescribing*. London: MHRA

Medicines for Human Use (Prescribing)(Miscellaneous Amendments) Order SI 2006 No 915

National Health Service (Miscellaneous Amendments Relating to Independent Prescribing) Regulations 2006 SI 2006 No 913 National Health Service (Primary Medical Services) Miscellaneous Amendments) Regulations SI 2005 No 893; The Medicines for Human Use (Prescribing) Order SI 2005 No 765

Nursing and Midwifery Council (2006) *Standards of Proficiency for Nurse* and *Midwife Prescribers*. NMC London

Nursing and Midwifery Council (2008) *Standards for Medicine Management* NMC London

Prescription Only Medicines (Human Use) Order 1977 SI 1997/1830

Prescription Only Medicines (Human Use) Amendment Order Statutory Instrument 2002 No 549

Statutory Instrument Prescription Only Medicines 1994 No 3050

CHAPTER 14

Complementary therapies

> **Box 14.1 Situation**
> Noel was a pain control nurse who, with his colleagues, provided a specialist service to the district hospital, being brought in by the wards and departments to assist in advising on pain management. In addition to his nursing qualification, he had also studied acupuncture and was able to offer an acupuncture service to the patients. Following one course of treatment, a patient complained that a needle had caused paralysis to her arm and she stated that she would sue the trust for compensation. What is the legal position of Noel?

Introduction

The popularity and growth in use of complementary and alternative therapies over recent years is a remarkable phenomenon. A *Complementary Medicine Information Pack for Primary Care* has been sponsored by the Department of Health and is available on its website (www.dh.gov.uk). The pack was initiated after a survey found that one in four adults would use alternative therapies at some point in their lives. The Health Education Authority (1995) has published an A to Z guide which covers 60 therapies.

The House of Lords Select Committee on Science and Technology held an inquiry into complementary medicine. It reported in November 2000 and recommended that there should be regulations of complementary and alternative medicines (CAM) and there should be further research to evaluate their effectiveness. It divided such therapies into three groups:

1. Professionally organised therapies, where there is some scientific evidence of their success, although seldom of the highest quality, and there are recognised systems for treatment and training of practitioners. This group includes acupuncture, chiropractic herbal medicine, homeopathy and osteopathy.
2. Complementary medicines where evidence that they work is generally lacking but which are used as an adjunct rather than a replacement for conventional therapies, so that lack of evidence may not matter so much. Included in this group are the Alexander technique, aromatherapy, nutritional medicine, hypnotherapy and Bach and other flower remedies.

3. Techniques that offer diagnosis as well as treatment, but for which scientific evidence is almost completely lacking. This group cannot be supported and includes naturopathy, crystal therapy, kinesiology, radionics, dowsing and iridology.

The Select Committee of the House of Lords considered that some remedies such as acupuncture and aromatherapy should be available on the NHS and NHS patients should have wider access to osteopathy and chiropractic.

The British Medical Association, at its conference in 2000, also recommended that acupuncture should be available on the NHS.

Complementary and alternative therapy use

The practitioner in pain management needs to be aware of two separate issues which may arise in the use of complementary therapies. One is the legal implications if he himself becomes a practitioner of such therapies as Noel in *Box 14.1*. The other is the legal significance of a patient utilising complementary therapies in addition to the orthodox treatments provided under the NHS. This latter situation shall be considered first.

Patients using complementary therapies

Practitioners in pain management (here referred to as pain practitioners) may discover quite by chance that their patients are also trying out various complementary or alternative therapies. There are possible dangers because certain orthodox treatments may be contraindicated if the patient is receiving other treatments. For example if a physiotherapist is assisting a patient who has chronic back pain, there may be conflicts with treatment provided by a chiropractic practitioner. It is advisable for the pain practitioner to obtain the patient's consent to contact the other practitioner in order to ensure that there are no conflicts between the different treatment plans. Should the patient refuse to give such consent, or refuse to allow records to be exchanged between the two practitioners, then the pain practitioner might have to advise the patient that because of potential dangers, he or she could not continue to treat the patient in ignorance of the plan being followed by the other practitioner.

It is essential that the pain practitioner is aware of the significance of the other treatments being given to the patient and acquires as much knowledge as possible about them.

The pain practitioner as complementary therapist

Where pain practitioners develop skills in a complementary therapy and wish to practise this as part of their NHS work, it is essential that the employer is aware of their intentions and gives approval for it. Without this approval, should harm result from negligent practice of the complementary therapy, the employer may be able to argue that this therapy was practised outside the course of employment and it is therefore not vicariously liable for it. (See *Chapter 4*.) Many NHS trusts now have a procedure for checking on the competence of an employee to practise a specific complementary therapy as part of his or her employment and for giving approval to that. It is preferable to obtain such approval in writing. Sometimes, an NHS trust may insist that all patients give consent before a complementary therapy is used upon them. A nurse who is skilled in aromatherapy, might consider that his or her skills could bring comfort to patients in the intensive care unit. However it is unlikely that consent could be obtained before the patient is placed on the ventilator, and therefore the nurse would be unable to provide aromatherapy for such patients. At the present time, until such therapies become part of orthodox medicine, it would not be possible to argue that they are in the best interests of a mentally incapacitated patient and could therefore be given to unconscious patients without their consent.

It is essential that the employee obtains the employer's consent to work privately on the premises. The following case concerned an occupational therapist who was conducting work as a private occupational therapist in the hospital, but the same principles would apply to an employee carrying out complementary therapies.

Mr Watling, an occupational therapist, who was forbidden to operate his private business was held to have been fairly dismissed (*Watling v Gloucestershire County Council Employment Tribunal*). He was warned not to engage in private work during his working week. He was observed by a manager seeing a private client during his lunch break and was dismissed for gross misconduct. He had ignored the warning and continued seeing private clients. He applied to an industrial tribunal and his dismissal was held by the tribunal to have been fair. He also failed in his appeal to the employment appeal tribunal. His defence that he was doing no more than taking an early lunch was rejected on the grounds that lunch hours are for lunch and not for seeing private patients. The employment appeal tribunal was satisfied that the employer had conducted a reasonable and fair enquiry into what had happened and that the decision of the industrial tribunal was beyond any sensible criticism.

Complementary and Natural Healthcare Council

The Prince's Foundation for Integrated Health set up a Federal Working Group which spent 12 months considering the formation of a new Council. Its report was published in February 2008. It recommended developing a federal structure for the voluntary self-regulation of complementary healthcare professions, i.e. a single regulatory body rather than a series of regulators for each complementary healthcare profession. At the time of writing a new body called the Complementary and Natural Healthcare Council (CNHC) has been established. It is made up of four elements:

- Federal Regulatory Council
- Profession Specific Boards
- Functional Boards
- Practice Advisory Panel.

CNHC has four main functions:

- To establish and maintain a voluntary register of complementary healthcare practitioners in the UK who meet its standards of competence and practice.
- To make the register of practitioners available to the general public and to educate them about the CNHC quality mark as a quality standard.
- To operate a robust process for handling complaints about registered practitioners.
- To work with professional bodies in the complementary healthcare field to further develop and improve standards of professional practice.

The CNHC describes itself as the national voluntary regulator for complementary healthcare practitioners. The members of the Council and the functional boards are lay people, appointed independently; each Profession Specific Board (one for each profession) has a lay chair and four registrants from the appropriate profession. Each Profession Specific Board selects one of its practitioner members to sit on the Practice Advisory Panel which provides a pool of expertise to support the Council. The report recommended robust procedures for handling complaints and fitness to practise issues, along with a code of conduct and ethics based on the code used by the Health Professions Council. The complementary healthcare professions that are, or have been, part of the Foundation for Integrated Health's regulation programme have developed, or are developing, the competencies necessary for entry to the Register. Full public and professional liability insurance will be mandatory, as will continuing professional development. The Federal Working Group has suggested that an independent, external organisation be invited to review the work of the Complementary and Natural Healthcare Council from time to time, to ensure that it remains fit for purpose and that it meets the needs of all who have an interest in its work. The Department of Health has provided start-up funding but the aim is for the Complementary and Natural Healthcare Council to be financed solely by registration fees. The Department of Health will also ensure that the principles underpinning professional regulation as set out in its White Paper *Trust, Assurance and Safety* (Department of Health, 2007) are implemented (see *Chapter 3*). The Council's register was in place in January 2009 with massage therapy and nutritional therapy; aromatherapy was added in May 2009 and over the next year further therapies including Alexander technique, Bowen technique, cranial therapy, homeopathy, naturopathy, reflexology, Reiki, Shiatsu, and Yoga will be included on the register.

To be eligible for registration, a practitioner must have undertaken a programme of education and training which meets, as a minimum, the National Occupational Standards for that profession/discipline or achieved competency to the same level by means of relevant experience and assessment. The Register can be checked on the CNHC's website (www.cnhc.org.uk). Criticism of the CNHC on the grounds that it was purporting to promote complementary therapies without any evidence of their efficacy was dismissed by the Government on the basis that it existed to protect the public by ensuring that registrants met a defined standard of practice.

A consultation on the Report to Ministers from the Department of Health Steering Group on the Statutory Regulation of Practitioners of Acupuncture, Herbal Medicine, Traditional Chinese Medicine and Other Traditional Medicine Systems Practised in the UK ended in November 2009. The Government response is currently awaited.

Application of the law to the situation in *Box 14.1*

Noel will have to establish that his work as an acupuncturist was carried out with the knowledge and therefore the express or implied consent of the employer. If he can establish this then he can argue that he was acting in the course of his employment in providing the acupuncture services. If it can be shown that the patient's paralysis was a reasonably foreseeable result of negligence on his part, then his employer would be vicariously liable for his negligence and would have to pay compensation to the patient. (It may of course be that the paralysis was not caused by the acupuncture needle, in which case the claimant would not succeed in an action for compensation, see *Chapter 4*). On the other hand if Noel is unable to show that he was acting in the course of employment, (this would be particularly so if he took payment from the patients and was acting as a self-employed practitioner in this work), then he is personally accountable for the harm which has been caused and would have to rely upon his own indemnity insurance cover. If he lacked such insurance cover, then his home and other possessions could be put at risk.

Conclusions

The implementation of the recommendations of the Select Committee of the House of Lords will lead to fundamental changes in how complementary and alternative therapies are viewed in relation to orthodox medicine and within the NHS. It is essential that pain practitioners who wish to practise in these fields are sure of their competence to do so and take steps to obtain the written agreement of their employer to use these therapies in addition to the skills from their registered professions. The future will see an increasing concern to obtain proof through random controlled trials that these non-orthodox treatments are effective.

Questions and exercises

1. Establish whether your employer has a check list and procedure to ensure the competence and approval for those employees who wish to practice complementary or alternative therapies.
2. How do you prove that you are competent in a complementary or alternative therapy?
3. Which complementary and alternative therapies, if any, do you consider should be available on the NHS and why?

References

Department of Health (2007) *Trust, Assurance and Safety: The Regulation of Health Professionals in the 21st Century*. White Paper Cmnd 7013. London: Department of Health

Health Education Authority (1995) *A-Z Guide on Complementary Therapies*. London: Health Education Authority

House of Lords Select Committee on Science and Technology (2000) *Sixth Report on Complementary and Alternative Medicine. Session 1999-2000*. London: House of Lords Select Committee on Science and Technology

Prince's Foundation for Integrated Health (2008) *A Federal Approach to Professionally-Led Voluntary Regulation for Complementary Healthcare: A plan for Action*. London: Prince's Foundation for Integrated Health

Watling v Gloucestershire County Council Employment Tribunal. EAT/868/94, 17 March 1995, 23 November 1994, Lexis transcript

CHAPTER 15

Scope of professional practice

> **Box 15.1 Situation**
> Marcus is a registered physiotherapist specialising in musculoskeletal problems. He would find it useful to prescribe a sedative to his patients before he treats them. At present he has to arrange for the patient to be written up for such medication by the doctor. He is seeking prescribing powers. What is the law?

Introduction

As the developments envisaged in the NHS Plan (Department of Health, 2000) have taken effect, so the significance of the original training of a registered practitioner counts for less than the post-registration training and experience. Many healthcare activities may be undertaken by practitioners from a variety of registered professions. The Government's plans for the new NHS as shown in *The New NHS – Modern Dependable* (Department of Health, 1997), in the document *Making a Difference* (Department of Health, 1999) and in the NHS Plan rely heavily upon a widened scope of practice for the nurse and other health professions. NHS Direct and walk-in clinics are run by nurses and provide an increasingly extensive and popular service. Standards and organisational issues are considered in *Chapter 17* of this book.

Statutory provisions

Unless an Act of Parliament or other statutory provision requires an activity to be undertaken by a specific health professional, then, provided the necessary training, experience and knowledge are acquired so that the activity can be undertaken competently, any registered health professional can undertake that activity. There are very few statutes which require activities to be performed only by a practitioner of specified registered profession. One of these is the Mental Health Act 1983. The detention of a patient under Section 2 or 3 of the Mental Health Act 1983 must be based on the recommendations of two registered medical practitioners. However other sections which have stipulated a specific health professional to perform specified functions have changed.

For example under section 5(2) of the 1983 Act only the registered medical practitioner treating the patient or a registered medical practitioner nominated by the former could detain an informal patient for up to 72 hours. However this duty, as a result of the Mental Health Act 2007 can now be undertaken by the approved clinician responsible for the patient's treatment. Registered professionals other than doctors, such as social workers, nurses, occupational therapists and psychologists, are eligible to become approved clinicians. The approved clinician can now undertake statutory duties under the Act which could formerly only be performed by a registered medical practitioner.

Another example of legislation stipulating a specific health professional is the Abortion Act 1967 which requires an approved termination to be carried out by a registered medical practitioner. However, the House of Lords interpreted this as meaning that the doctor responsible for the termination when prostaglandins were being administered could supervise its being carried out by a nurse (*Royal College of Nursing of the UK v Department of Health and Social Security* [1981]). As Lord Diplock said in the House of Lords:

> *The doctor need not do everything with his own hands; the subsection's requirements were satisfied when the treatment was one prescribed by a registered medical practitioner carried out in accordance with his directions and of which he remained in charge throughout.*

The Medicines Act 1968, as we saw in *Chapter 13*, is also specific as to which named professions could undertake activities under the Act, but Section 63 of the Health and Social Care Act 2001 has extended the provisions of Section 58 of the Medicines Act 1968 to enable other registered health practitioners to have prescribing powers.

Prescribing powers

The extension of prescribing powers (see *Chapter 13*) to additional professions has had a major impact upon role definition. Regulations identifying those practitioners who could prescribe against an agreed protocol under a patient group direction came into force on 9 August 2000 (Prescription only Medicines [Human Use] Amendment Order 2000). The regulations clarifying independent and supplementary prescribers and the conditions of their prescribing have greatly enhanced the role of pain practitioners.

Other areas of role expansion

Other areas in which pain practitioners may develop their skills include:

• Triage of patients in accident and emergency departments.

- Nurse-led pain relief clinics, for example in acupuncture, transcutaneous electric nerve stimulation (TENS).
- Spinal cord implant clinics.
- Transcribing from group protocols onto the ward drug charts (see *Chapter 13*).
- Audit on records for pain assessment and management (see *Chapter 19*).

Conditions for developing the scope of professional practice

Same standard of care

Where an activity is undertaken by a different professional than the one who would normally undertake that activity, the law requires that the same standard of the competent professional as per the Bolam Test is followed. It is no defence to argue that a person with less training or experience carried out that activity, if harm to the patient occurs. The patient is entitled to expect that he or she would receive the reasonable standard of care whoever is undertaking that activity. In 1992 the UKCC laid down principles for the safe development of the scope of professional practice, which are relevant to all healthcare professionals. They are shown in *Box 15.2*.

Box 15.2 Principles for adjusting the scope of professional practice

The registered nurse, midwife or health visitor:
- must be satisfied that each aspect of practice is directed to meeting the needs and serving the interests of the patient or client;
- must endeavour always to achieve, maintain and develop knowledge, skill and competence to respond to those needs and interests;
- must honestly acknowledge any limits of personal knowledge and skill and take steps to remedy any relevant deficits in order effectively and appropriately to meet the needs of patients and clients;
- must ensure that any enlargement or adjustment of the scope of personal professional practice must be achieved without compromising or fragmenting existing aspects of professional practice and care and that requirements of the Council's Code of Professional Conduct are satisfied throughout the whole area of practice;
- must recognise and honour the direct or indirect personal accountability borne for all aspects of professional practice; and
- must, in serving the interests of patients and clients and the wider interests of society, avoid any inappropriate delegation to others which compromises those interests.

Subsequently the Nursing and Midwifery Council (NMC), which replaced the UKCC, provided its own guidance on expanding the scope of practice which is contained in its Code of Conduct published in 2008. Under the requirement to provide a high standard of care at all times, the NMC places the following duty upon registrants:

- You must have the knowledge and skills for safe and effective practice when working without direct supervision.
- You must recognise and work within the limits of your competence.
- You must keep your knowledge and skills up to date throughout your working life.
- You must take part in appropriate learning and practice activities that maintain and develop your competence and performance.

The latter requirement that the registrant must take part in appropriate training and practice activities that maintain and develop competence and performance contrasts with the right under the former concept of the extended role of the nurse whereby the nurse could refuse to undertake training to develop the scope of her practice. This is no longer an option. If the appropriate training is offered and the necessary resources provided to implement the developed scope of practice, then the nurse would be required to undertake the training and the expanded role.

Application of the law to the situation in *Box 15.1*

Marcus may be able to agree with the doctors treating his patients, that a patient group direction should be drawn up in accordance with the requirements as shown in *Box 13.2* in *Chapter 13*, which would enable him to give appropriate medication before treating his patients. He would need to follow the principles laid down in *Box 15.2* to ensure that he is competent to undertake this activity safely. He may also be able to undertake the training to establish himself as an independent or dependent practitioner in his particular field of work and be recognised as having the wider prescribing powers permitted under the law.

Conclusion

In its 1997 report *Anaesthesia under Examination*, the Audit Commission made significant recommendations on anaesthetic and pain management services and suggested that there was considerable scope for the role expansion of many of the different professional groups that work in theatres. The Report illustrates how problems can arise when inter-disciplinary teamworking breaks down. It puts forward practical suggestions on how NHS trusts can improve anaesthetic and pain relief services.

The protection of the patient is the competence of the individual practitioner caring for the patient. That practitioner must work within his or her field of competence, acknowledging any gaps in knowledge and expertise, and ensure that the necessary additional training, supervised practice and experience are obtained. Major developments can be expected in the next few years and it is essential that there are on-going multi-disciplinary discussions to ensure co-ordination of who is doing what, and when, in patient care and particularly in pain management.

Questions and exercises

1. In what ways do you consider that the scope of your professional practice could be developed?
2. How would you determine your competence to undertake any specific expanded role activity?
3. How can professionals ensure that there is co-ordination when several different professionals are able to undertake the same activities?

References

Audit Commission (1997) *Anaesthesia under Examination. The Efficiency and Effectiveness of Anaesthesia and Pain Relief Services in England and Wales*. London: Audit Commission

Department of Health (1997) *The New NHS – Modern Dependable*. London: HMSO

Department of Health (1999) *Making a Difference: The new NHS*. London: Department of Health

Department of Health (2000) *The NHS Plan: A Plan for Investment, a Plan for Reform*. London: Department of Health

Nursing and Midwifery Council (2008) *The Code: Standards of Conduct, Performance and Ethics for Nurses and Midwives*. London: NMC

Prescription only Medicines (Human Use) Amendment Order 2000 SI 2000 No 1917

Royal College of Nursing of the UK v Department of Health and Social Security [1981] AC 800; 1981 1 All ER 545

CHAPTER 16

Health and safety and consumer protection

> **Box 16.1 Situation**
> Serena was a staff nurse on the surgical ward and was administering post-operative analgesia to a patient when the needle broke as she was injecting. The tip of the needle was lost in the patient and could only be retrieved under a local anaesthetic. The patient is threatening to bring an action for compensation for the additional pain and suffering which she has undergone. What is the legal situation?

Introduction

Health and safety laws that protect the health and safety of employees, patients and the general public derive from many statutory and common law sources but the principle legislation is the Health and Safety at Work Act 1974 (HASWA) and the statutory instruments made under it. Section 2 places a duty on the employer to take reasonable care of the health, safety and welfare of its employees, and Section 3 places a duty on the employer to all those whose health or safety may be affected by its enterprise. Under Section 7 each employee has a duty to take reasonable care of the health and safety of him or herself and others and to co-operate with the employer in obeying health and safety laws. These statutory duties are enforced by way of criminal proceedings by the Health and Safety Executive and its inspectors. These statutory duties are paralleled by duties under the contract of employment under which the employer has an implied duty to take reasonable care for the health and safety of the employee and the employee a duty to obey the reasonable instructions of the employer; and by the laws of negligence, where (as we have seen in *Chapter 4*) a duty of care is owed to patients and others. Other statutory provisions cover the liability of the occupier to visitors (Occupier's Liability Act 1957) and to trespassers (Occupier's Liability Act 1984), the regulations relating to substances hazardous to health, the reporting of incidents of disease and the medical devices regulations. These are considered in more detail in the author's law books for nurses, midwives, physiotherapists and occupational therapists (see Dimond, 2004).

Relevance of health and safety laws to pain practitioners

Health and safety laws are relevant to pain practitioners whatever their registered profession. They need to have an understanding of the laws that apply to them and from whom they can obtain further information. For example, many pain practitioners may be involved in manual handling; assisting a patient into a more comfortable position may not be lifting, but would come within the definition of manual handling. The pain practitioner needs to have an understanding of how such an action can be undertaken safely and the basic legal requirements of the Manual Handling Regulations. One example of a statutory provision that will be taken to indicate the relevance of these laws to pain practitioners will be the Management of Health and Safety in the Workplace Regulations.

Management of Health and Safety in the Workplace Regulations 1999

These regulations require each employer to undertake a suitable and sufficient assessment of the risks to the health and safety of his or her employees. Suitable and sufficient are not defined within the regulations, but the approved code of practice and guidance gives practical advice on how to carry out a risk assessment (Health and Safety Commission, 1999; 2000).

Medical devices regulations

Almost all the equipment used by pain practitioners would come within the definition of a medical device. The definition used by the Medical Devices Agency, now incorporated within the Medicines and Healthcare Products Regulatory Agency (MHRA), is based upon the European Directive definition (93/42/EEC):

> *Any instrument, apparatus, material or other article, whether used alone or in combination, including the software necessary for its proper application, intended by the manufacturer to be used for human beings for the purpose of:*
> - *diagnosis, prevention, monitoring, treatment or alleviation of disease;*
> - *diagnosis, monitoring, treatment, alleviation of or compensation for an injury or handicap;*
> - *investigation, replacement or modification of the anatomy or of a physiological process;*
> - *control of contraception;*
> *and which does not achieve its principal intended action in or on the human*

body by pharmacological, immunological or metabolic means, but which may be assisted in its function by such means.

Pain practitioners must ensure that they are aware of any warning notices that are issued by the Medicines and Healthcare Products Regulatory Agency. Warning notices and helpful information is available on its website (www.mhra.gov.uk). They must also ensure that they are aware of the procedure for the notification of any defects and who is their liaison officer for the purposes of the Medical Devices Agency (MDA) regulations.

National Patient Safety Agency (NPSA)

The NPSA was established in 2001 to run the mandatory reporting system for logging all failures, mistakes, errors and near misses across the health services (Department of Health, 2001a). The Department of Health's (2001b) publication *Building a Safer NHS for Patients* sets out details of the scheme together with recommendations for an improved system for handling investigations and inquiries across the NHS. The NPSA's website (www.npsa.gov.uk) provides information about product safety and initiatives to reduce harm resulting from hazards and risks. It aims to ensure that the NHS learns from all adverse incidents that occur across the country.

Consumer Protection Act 1987

The Consumer Protection Act 1987 enables a claim to be brought where harm has occurred as a result of a defect in a product. It is a form of strict liability in that negligence by the supplier or manufacturer does not have to be established. The claimant will however have to show that there was a defect. The supplier can rely upon a defence colloquially known as 'state of the art', i.e. that the state of scientific and technical knowledge at the time the goods were supplied was not such that the producer of products of that kind might be expected to have discovered the defect. The claim is brought against the manufacturer or supplier of the goods. A successful claim was brought in March 1993 (Dimond, 1993) when Simon Garratt was awarded £1400 against the manufacturers of a pair of surgical scissors that broke during an operation on his knee, with the blade being left embedded. A second operation was required to remove it. Had he relied upon the law of negligence to obtain compensation he would have had to show that the manufacturers were in breach of the duty of care which they owed to him.

Patients who had contracted hepatitis C from blood and blood products used in blood transfusions brought a case under the Consumer Protection Act 1987 and succeeded (*A and Others v National Blood Authority and Another*). This decision may well lead to greater use of the Consumer Protection Act

1987 where personal injuries are caused as a result of defective products, since negligence does not have to be established under the Consumer Protection Act 1987, only that there was a defect in the product that has caused the harm.

Application of the law to the situation in *Box 16.1*

The patient has many possible causes of action in the situation described in *Box 16.1*. There may well be a possible claim for negligence against the employer of Serena who is vicariously liable for her negligence. It would have to be shown that Serena was in breach of the duty of care which she owed to the patient. There may however be considerable difficulties in establishing that Serena was in breach of the duty of care. Alternatively, and probably more effectively, the patient could bring an action against the suppliers or manufacturers of the needles. The patient would need to be given details of the product from the hospital: the name and address of the manufacturers or suppliers and if possible the batch numbers. If the hospital is unable to provide this information, then it becomes the supplier for the purposes of the Consumer Protection Act 1987. Serena must ensure that notification of the defect is made to the hospital liaison officer who is in contact with the Medicines and Healthcare Products Regulatory Agency. In addition a report should be made to the National Patient Safety Agency.

Conclusions

It will be evident that this chapter has barely touched the surface of the vast body of legislation and case law that applies to health and safety and the practitioner is referred to relevant works cited in the further reading section on p. 177. Regular contact with the NHS trust health and safety officer would ensure that the practitioner keeps up to date.

Questions and exercises

1. Check the record of accidents that have taken place over the past month and consider the extent to which these could have been avoided.
2. Observe your practice for a week and the types of equipment and instruments that would come within the definition of a medical device. Ensure that you regularly receive notifications from the MHRA.
3. How do the Management of Health and Safety Regulations apply to your work?

References

A and Others v National Blood Authority and Another. The Times Law Report 4 April 2001

Department of Health (2001a) *National patient safety agency to be launched.* Press release. London: Department of Health

Department of Health (2001b) *Building a Safer NHS for Patients.* London: Department of Health

Dimond BC (1993) Protecting the consumer. *Nursing Standard* 7(4): 18–19

Dimond BC (2004) *Legal Aspects of Heath and Safety.* London: Quay Books

Health and Safety Commission (1999) *Management of Health and Safety at Work Regulations.* London: HSC

Health and Safety Commission (2000) *Approved Code of Practice and Guidance.* London: HSC

CHAPTER 17

Standards and organisational issues

> ### Box 17.1 Situation
> Mustafa suffered considerable pain whilst he was in hospital and was appalled to discover that there was no pain management service provided by the hospital. He understood that the trust board was under a statutory duty to lay down and monitor standards of quality and was considering suing the board for its failure to provide a reasonable service and fulfil its statutory obligations.

Introduction

In *Chapter 15* we considered developments in the scope of professional practice in the light of Government plans as shown in the White Paper *The New NHS – Modern Dependable* (Department of Health, 1997), in the document *Making a Difference* (Department of Health, 1999) and in the NHS Plan (Department of Health, 2000). Legislation implementing these plans is to be found in the Health Act 1999, the Health and Social Care Act 2001, the NHS Reform and Health Care Professions Act 2002, Health and Social Care (Community Health and Standards) Act 2003, the NHS Redress Act 2006 and the Health and Social Care Act 2008 and the Health Act 2009. Over recent years the following have been initiated: the National Institute for Clinical Excellence (now the National Institute for Health and Clinical Excellence), the Commission for Health Improvement (followed by the Commission for Health Audit and Inspection which was merged into the Care Quality Commission in April 2009), the National Service Frameworks, the National Patient Safety Agency and many others.

Clinical governance

One of the most important initiatives was the introduction of the concept of clinical governance. It derives from the statutory duty under Section 18 of the Health Act 1999 which is shown in *Box 17.2*.

The duty falls primarily upon the chief executive of each health authority and NHS trust.

> ### Box 17.2 Section 18 Health Act 1999
> It is the duty of each Health Authority, Primary Care Trust and NHS Trust
> to put and keep in place arrangements for the purpose of monitoring and
> improving the quality of health care which it provides to individuals.

The result of this statutory duty is that NHS Trust Boards and their chief officers are responsible for the standard of clinical care within the organisation. If they fail to ensure that reasonable standards of care are in place, then the board and its chairman and chief officers can be replaced by the Secretary of State. As a consequence of this power greater freedom has been granted to those NHS trusts whose hospitals have reached high standards in the league tables and the management of poor performers has been taken over (Department of Health, 2002a). In 2002 the zero-rated trusts were given three months to show clear signs of improvement. Those that failed to show such improvements had their management taken over by successful managers from other trusts or from the private sector (Department of Health, 2002b). As a consequence of the Health and Social Care (Community Health and Standards) Act 2003 NHS Foundation Trusts were set up which have enjoyed greater freedom than the other NHS trusts and come under the aegis of a regulator.

Section 46 of the Health and Social Care (Community Health and Standards) Act 2003 gave power to the Secretary of State to prepare and publish statements of standards in relation to the provision of healthcare by and for English NHS bodies and cross-border Strategic Health Authorities (SHAs). These provisions were re-enacted in Section 45 of the Health and Social Care Act 2008.

Under Section 45(1) the Secretary of State may prepare and publish statements of standards in relation to the provision of NHS care and under 45(2) the Secretary of State must keep the standards under review and may publish amended statements whenever the Secretary of State considers it appropriate. In addition the Secretary of State may direct a person:

(a) to prepare a draft statement of standards for the purposes of subsection (1), submit it to the Secretary of State for approval and publish it in the form approved or modified by the Secretary of State;
(b) to keep standards under review for the purposes of subsection (2) and, whenever the person considers it appropriate, submit a draft amended statement to the Secretary of State for approval and publish it in the form approved or modified by the Secretary of State.

Under Section 45(4) the Secretary of State must consult such persons as the Secretary of State considers appropriate:

(a) before publishing a statement under subsection (1) or approving a statement under subsection (3)(a);

(b) before publishing under subsection (2), or approving under subsection (3) (b), any amended statement which in the opinion of the Secretary of State effects a substantial change in the standards.

The Care Quality Commission has the power to inspect NHS organisations against these standards.

National Institute of Health and Clinical Excellence (NICE)

This statutory body was established on 1 April 1999 to promote clinical and cost effectiveness. The then Secretary of State stated that its task would be to abolish postcode variation in the country, so that there would be national standards for the provision of healthcare, such as medicines. One of the functions of NICE is to issue clinical guidelines and clinical audit methodologies and information on good practice. NICE has a major role to play in the setting of standards of practice, by disseminating the results of research of what is proved to be clinically effective, research-based practice. It is essential that pain practitioners are aware of the reports and recommendations of NICE. It does not follow that they will automatically become binding on practitioners, since practitioners will still have to use their professional discretion in deciding whether the guidelines are appropriate for the care and treatment of the individual patient. However if practitioners fail to follow the guidelines, they would have to give clear reasons why they were not appropriate for the circumstances of that individual patient. It is likely that as its work progresses more of its recommendations whether on medications or clinical procedures will relate to pain management. Claimants may be able to show that there has been a breach of the duty of care which has caused harm by establishing that NICE guidelines were ignored.

Care Quality Commission (CQC)

Sections 19 to 24 of the Health Act 1999 establish the Commission for Health Improvement and sets out its functions and powers. This was replaced by the Commission for Health Audit and Inspection which, together with the Commission for Social Care Inspection and the Mental Health Act Commission, was absorbed into the Care Quality Commission in April 2009. The Care Quality Commission is a body corporate, i.e. it can sue and be sued on its own account. It undertakes inspections of NHS trusts, health authorities and primary care trusts, private hospitals and care organisations. Information relating to its functions and activities can be obtained on its website (www. cqc.org.uk).

National Service Frameworks (NSF)

NSFs have been set up for several specialties including mental health, coronary heart disease, cancer care and older peoples' services, diabetes and for children, young people and maternity services. Pain management may eventually have its own NSF or be included in several different frameworks. The NSF sets minimum standards to be achieved across the specific specialty and could become a major justification for the redistribution of resources. For example in pain management, if pain practitioners were aware that an NSF recommended that in each hospital there should be a central service for pain management advice and treatment, then this could be used as justification for the allocation of resources for such a service.

Kennedy Report

The report on paediatric heart surgery in Bristol (*Bristol Royal Infirmary Learning from Bristol: The report of the public inquiry into children's heart surgery at the Bristol Royal Infirmary 1984–1995*) has made significant recommendations for a fundamental change in the relationship between patients and professionals within the NHS. Implementation of these recommendations should ensure that there is openness and honesty between professionals and patients and, where concerns are raised, these are dealt with honestly. Patients should be told of untoward events.

Application of the law to the situation in *Box 17.1*

Mustafa may well have an action in negligence if he can show that there was a failure to follow the reasonable standard of care in controlling his pain. If he can establish that the ward staff did not follow basic principles of pain management and as a consequence he suffered additional harm, then he may have grounds for suing the trust for its vicarious liability for the negligence of its staff. Mustafa may be able to argue that there has been a breach of his rights under Article 3 of the European Convention on Human Rights since he has suffered inhuman and degrading treatment. He may also have an action for breach of the direct liability of the trust to him for its failure to establish a safe system for pain management in its hospital. This latter course of action would be more problematic in its success. It is unlikely that the courts would see that an individual patient had a right to sue a trust for breach of its statutory duty under Section 18 of the Health Act 1999. Usually breach of a statutory duty is not open as a cause of action to a claimant if there are other remedies. In this statute other remedies would include the right of the Secretary of State to remove the trust board, or for the claimant to pursue a complaint against the trust. The handling of complaints is considered in the next chapter.

Conclusions

The significant changes that have taken place in the NHS over the past few years have placed considerable pressures upon practitioners to be aware of recommendations, advice guidelines, procedures and protocols issued by the new institutions. Ignorance of recommended practice would be no defence to a practitioner if such advice had become incorporated into the standards of the reasonable practitioner as set out in the Bolam Test.

Questions and exercises

1. Examine the extent to which NICE recommendations relate to pain management.
2. A Care Quality Commission inspection is due to take place in your trust over the next three months. What preparations would you make for such a visit and how would it help you ensure a high standard of care for your patients?
3. To what extent has the NSF for the care of cancer patients been implemented in your trust and how has it affected your practice?

References

Bristol Royal Infirmary. Learning from Bristol: The report of the public inquiry into children's heart surgery at the Bristol Royal Infirmary 1984–1995. Command Paper CM 5207 July 2001. Available from: http://www.bristol-inquiry.org.uk/

Department of Health (1997) *The New NHS –Modern Dependable.* London: HMSO

Department of Health (1999) *Making a Difference The new NHS.* London: Department of Health

Department of Health (2000) *The NHS Plan: A plan for investment, a plan for reform.* London: Department of Health

Department of Health (2002a) *Milburn announces radical decentralisation of NHS control.* Press Release 2002/0022. London: Department of Health

Department of Health (2002b) Press release 2002/0069. London: Department of Health

CHAPTER 18

Complaints and patient representation

Box 18.1 Situation

Sunny was admitted to hospital for the birth of her first child, although she had hoped to have had a home birth. Subsequently she complained that she had been given an epidural without her consent and had wanted to have minimum intervention. She asked the midwife for her complaint to be investigated.

Introduction

The Hospital Complaints Act 1985 sought to ensure that in each hospital there was an effective procedure for dealing with complaints by patients and their representatives and was followed by guidance recommending that the complaints machinery should also be extended to community health services. In 1994 the recommendations of the Wilson Committee (Department of Health, 1994) for dealing with hospital and primary care complaints were implemented in the establishment in 1996 of a complaints procedure. Subsequently in the NHS Plan (Department of Health, 2000) the Government stated that it was to establish a National Patient Safety Agency to set up a full mandatory reporting scheme for adverse healthcare events (see *Chapter 17*), an improved professional regulatory mechanism for doctors and other health professionals (see *Chapter 5*), and a new patient advocacy service.

Chapter 10 of the NHS Plan sets out the strategy for implementing significant changes for patient care. These include:

* More information for patients.
* Greater patient choice.
* Patients' advocates and advisers in every hospital.
* Redress over cancelled operations.
* Patients' forums and citizens' panels in every trust.
* New national panel to advise on major reorganisations of hospitals.

- Stronger regulation of professional standards.

These changes, some of which needed legislative provision, have been implemented, together with a new complaints system introduced in 2004.

Background to the Complaints Procedure 2004

Complaints procedure

The effectiveness of the complaints system established in 1996 was reviewed in 2001 and in the light of the results of that research the Department of Health (2001a) published a document suggesting a number of ways to improve the procedure. The Department of Health also issued a consultation document (2001b) on which feedback was invited. In 2003 the Department of Health's publication, *NHS Complaints Reform: Making things right* noted the following criticisms of the 1996 complaints procedure:

- It is unclear how to pursue complaints and concerns.
- There is often a delay in responding when concerns arise.
- Too often there is a negative attitude to concerns expressed.
- Complaints seem not to get a fair hearing.
- Patients do not get the support they need when they want to complain.
- The independent review stage does not have the credibility it needs.
- The process does not provide the redress the patients want.
- There does not seem to be any systematic processes for using feedback from complaints to drive improvements in services.

The aims of the 2003 reforms to the complaints procedure were to establish clear national standards and accountabilities, to achieve devolution to clinicians and managers backed up by independent scrutiny and flexibility and to ensure that patients can choose how they wish to pursue their concerns and have the support they need to help them do so.

The Department of Health recommended that there should be:

- Increasing support and information for people who make complaints through local patient advice and liaison services and independent complaints and advice services (see below).
- Patient feedback and customer care and training for NHS staff, including board members, to improve the way people are dealt with to help resolve complaints quickly.
- Subject to legislation, placing responsibility for independent complaints review with the Commission for Healthcare Audit and Inspection (CHAI), known as the Healthcare Commission.

The Complaints Procedure 2004

The new complaints procedure envisaged three stages similar to the procedure following the Wilson report: local, intermediate and Health Service Ombudsman, but the intermediate stage was made more independent by its being placed upon the Healthcare Commission. Regulations were brought into force on 30 July 2004 (National Health Service [Complaints] Regulations 2004) on a new complaints system and amended in 2006 (National Health Service [Complaints] Regulations 2006). The Regulations can be accessed on the website of the Office of Public Sector Information (www.opsi.gov.uk). Guidance is provided by the Department of Health on both sets of regulations and is available on its website (www.dh.gov.uk/). From the 1 April 2009 the independent stage of complaints investigation, which was carried out by the Healthcare Commission (since abolished and replaced by the Care Quality Commission), was taken over by the Health Service Ombudsman thus turning the three-stage complaints procedure into a two-stage complaints procedure.

The regulations cover:

- The nature and scope of arrangements for the handling and consideration of complaints.
- The handling and consideration of complaints by NHS bodies.
- The handling and consideration of complaints by the Healthcare Commission (Care Quality Commission). (This stage was subsequently abolished in April 2009 and complainants who are dissatisfied can apply to the Health Service Ombudsman for further investigation.)
- Publicity, monitoring and annual reports.

The regulations require each NHS body and each primary care trust to make arrangements for the handling of complaints in accordance with the regulations.

The arrangements must be accessible and such as to ensure that the complaints are dealt with speedily and efficiently, and that complainants are treated courteously and sympathetically and as far as possible involved in decisions about how their complaints are handled and considered.

The arrangements must be in writing with a copy given free of charge to any person who requests it.

Amendments were made to the Regulations in 2006 (National Health Service [Complaints] Amendment Regulations 2006) to facilitate the transfer of complaints which relate to social services, extending the persons who can be appointed as complaints managers (the complaints manager does not have to be an employee of the NHS body and can be appointed for more than one NHS body), changing the time limit for response to a complaint and broadening the remit of the Healthcare Commission in relation to complaints about NHS Foundation Trusts. (This second stage of the complaints procedure was abolished in April 2009 – and complainants can now apply to the Health Service Ombudsman.)

A primary care provider (and this includes pharmacists, ophthalmic opticians, dentists, GPs and primary care trusts) must ensure that a complaints procedure is in place. A complex complaint is one that relates to several different NHS bodies or local authority or primary care providers or is already subject to a concurrent investigation. If the NHS trust or primary care trust arranges for the provision of services through an independent provider, it is required to ensure that the independent provider has arrangements in place for the handling of complaints in accordance with the regulations.

Criticisms of the 2004 Complaints Procedure

In October 2007 the Healthcare Commission (since April 2009 the Care Quality Commission) published its first audit on how the NHS trusts handled complaints. This is available on the Care Quality Commission website (www. cqc.org.uk/). It found considerable variation in how complaints were handled across the country. Amongst its criticisms were:

- More needs to be done to make the complaints systems open and accessible, especially for those with learning disabilities and from minority ethnic communities.
- People who complain should be confident that their care will not suffer.
- Trusts should use complaints' data to inform decision making.
- Whilst there is no one-size-fits-all approach to investigating complaints, a common approach would improve risk management of complaints and manage the expectations of complainants.
- There are no nationally available standard tools and resources such as case studies, checklists and training aids for staff.

The Patients Association has also made criticisms of the complaints system, calling for NHS trust boards to be publicly accountable for an open, transparent and timely resolution of complaints (Rose, 2008). Following a report by the Healthcare Commission into the deaths and A & E failures at Mid Staffordshire NHS Foundation Trust in March 2009 (available on the website of the Care Quality Commission, www.cqc.org.uk/), the Department of Health announced that all hospitals in England would have to report the number and details of complaints that they receive and they would be published on the NHS website (Rose, 2009).

Patient Advocacy and Liaison Service (PALS)

The NHS Plan (Department of Health, 2000) proposed the establishment of a Patient Advocacy and Liaison Service (PALS) in every major hospital with an annual national budget of around £10 million. A new patient advocacy team, usually situated in the main reception areas of hospitals, acts as a welcoming point for patients and carers and a clearly identifiable information point. Patient advocates act as an independent facilitator to handle patient and family concerns, with direct access to the chief executive and the power to negotiate immediate solutions. They work with other organisations, such as the Citizens Advice Bureau.

Patients' Forums

Patients' Forums were set up in every NHS trust and primary care trust to provide direct input from patients about how local NHS services are run. Patients had a direct representation on every NHS Trust Board. The representatives were elected by the Patients' Forum. The Forum was supported by each PALS and had the right to visit and inspect any aspect of the trust's care at any time. In 2006 the Department of Health published its report *A Stronger Local Voice* which announced that Patients' Forums in England were to be abolished and replaced by local authority run Local Involvement Networks (LINKs) under the Local Government and Public Involvement in Health Act 2007. (See below.)

Commission for Public and Patient Involvement in Health

In accordance with the strategy set out in the NHS Plan (Department of Health, 2000) the Commission for Patient and Public Involvement in Health (CPPIH) was established under Section 20 of the NHS Reform and Health Care Professions Act 2002 in January 2003. Its functions, set out in Section 20(2) of the 2002 Act, included advising the Secretary of State about arrangements for public involvement in and consultation about matters relating to the health service in England and the provision of independent advocacy services. It was abolished in 2008 when the Local Government and Public Involvement in Health Act 2007, which set up Local Involvement Networks, came into force (see below).

Local Involvement Networks (LINKs)

Part 14 of the Local Government and Public Involvement in Health Act 2007 established Local Involvement Networks for health and social services. Under

Section 221 each local authority is required to make contractual arrangements for the purpose of ensuring that there are means by which specified activities can be carried on in the area. The activities specified include:

• Promoting and supporting the involvement of people in the commissioning, provision and scrutiny of local care services.
• Enabling people to monitor for the purposes of their consideration of specified matters (standard of provision of local care services, how they could be improved and whether and how they ought to be improved) and to review for those purposes the commissioning and provision of local care services.
• Obtaining the views of people about their needs for, and their experience of, local care services, and
• Making these views known and making reports on recommendations about how local care services could or ought to be improved, to persons responsible for commissioning, providing, managing or scrutinising local care services.

Local care services means services provided as part of the health services and social services of a local authority. The Local Involvement Network (LINK) which results from these arrangements cannot include a local authority or health services organisation. The service providers must allow entry by LINKs. The LINK must provide an annual report which contains matters to be specified by the Secretary of State and sent to the local authority and NHS organisations in the area. Regulations on LINKs came into force on 1 April 2008 (Local Involvement Networks Regulations S.I. 2008). As a consequence of this, the Patient Forums and the Commission for Public and Patient Involvement in Health were abolished. The Audit Commission and the Healthcare Commission reported in June 2008 that the reforms, costing £1 billion to make the NHS more efficient and patient-friendly, have failed to have much impact.

The Department has asked the NHS Centre for Involvement (NCI) to provide ongoing help, advice and support to help LINKs get going. Since April 2008, a range of guides have been produced on different aspects of running LINKs. Examples include: setting up a governance structure and setting a work programme. LINKs representatives have the right to enter certain publicly funded health and care facilities. A code of conduct has been published by the NHS Centre for Involvement to ensure that visits are proportionate, reasonable and do not impact on the rights of people who use services. The Department of Health has recommended both LINKs and providers to use this guidance.

The NHS Reform and Healthcare Professions Act abolished Community Health Councils in England but they have been retained in Wales.

Application of the law to the situation in *Box 18.1*

It is advisable for Sunny to be asked to put her complaint in writing, but even if it is just a complaint by word of mouth it should be properly investigated. Under the present scheme for handling complaints, there would be an attempt to resolve it at a local level. There would be a thorough investigation in which the midwife would be asked for a detailed account of what happened, the condition of Sunny and her requests. Following this investigation the results would be reported to Sunny. If Sunny were not satisfied with the response she would have the right to apply to the Health Service Commissioner, the Ombudsman, for an independent investigation into her complaint. In the light of the serious criticisms of the 2004 Complaints procedure by the Healthcare Commission, the Patient's Association and the National Audit Office, it is likely that there will once again be significant changes to the procedure. Sunny may find that she has a right of legal redress because of her complaint, since the investigation may reveal that she has an action for trespass to her person and/or an action for negligence in her care which has caused her harm. If this is revealed during the complaints process, Sunny may well have to decide whether to pursue the complaints process or initiate litigation instead. Since a complaint about which the complainant has stated in writing that he or she intends to take legal proceedings is excluded from the present complaints procedure, Sunny might have to make a decision as to whether to follow the path of litigation or one of complaint. At the time of writing the NHS Redress Act 2006 has not been brought into force. When it is implemented, Sunny would be able to pursue her claim through an NHS Redress scheme.

Conclusions

It has proved difficult in recent years to set up a procedure for handling complaints which is effective, efficient and meets patients' needs. More changes are required in the light of recent criticisms of the current system. Pain practitioners who are confident in their practice will welcome improved communication between patients and professionals and see complaints as a means of improving their service to the patient. The effectiveness of the new Local Involvement Networks is still to be proved.

Questions and exercises

1. Examine complaints received over the past month. To what extent can lessons be learnt from these complaints and improvements put in hand?
2. What benefits do you consider a patient's representative could bring to the service that you provide?
3. How could you obtain effective feedback on the service that you give to patients?

References

Department of Health (1994) *Being Heard. The Report of a Review Committee Chaired by Professor Wilson on NHS Complaints Procedures*. London: Department of Health

Department of Health (2000) *The NHS Plan. A Plan for Investment, a Plan for Reform*. London: Department of Health

Department of Health (2001a) *The NHS Complaints Procedure: National Evaluation*. London: Department of Health

Department of Health (2001b) *Reforming the NHS Complaints Procedure: A Listening Document*. London: Department of Health

Department of Health (2003) *NHS Complaints Reform: Making Things Right*. London: Department of Health

Local Involvement Networks Regulations S.I. 2008 No 528

National Health Service (Complaints) Regulations 2004 SI 1768

National Health Service (Complaints) Amendment Regulations 2006 No 2084

Rose D (2008) 'Pointless' NHS complaints system to become less rigid. *The Times* 22 September

Rose D (2009) Hospitals will be forced to publish complaints details. *The Times* 1 May

Record keeping

Introduction

There are few statutory provisions which apply to standards and the nature of documentation in healthcare. Exceptions include regulations under the Mental Health Act 1983, which requires statutory documents to be kept for detention and consent to treatment, and under the Abortion Act 1967, which also specifies which particulars are statutorily required. Reporting of health and safety incidents is also required under the Reporting of Injuries, Diseases and Dangerous Occurrences Regulations (RIDDOR) 1995. Guidance on RIDDOR is provided by the Health and Safety Executive (HSE) and is available from its website (www.hse.gov.uk/riddor/). Apart from such exceptions the law relating to standards of record keeping derives from the common law in relation to the reasonable standard of professional practice and guidance issued by registration bodies and professional associations.

Basic principles

The basic principle on which standards of record keeping rest is the care of the patient. The Nursing and Midwifery Council (NMC) (2009) emphasised that good record keeping is an integral part of nursing and midwifery practice, and is essential to the provision of safe and effective care. It is not an optional extra to be fitted in if circumstances allow.

The NMC states that

Good record keeping, whether at an individual, team or organisational level, has many important functions. These include a range of clinical, administrative and educational uses such as:
- *helping to improve accountability*
- *showing how decisions related to patient care were made*
- *supporting the delivery of services*
- *supporting effective clinical judgements and decisions*
- *supporting patient care and communications*
- *making continuity of care easier*
- *providing documentary evidence of services delivered*
- *promoting better communication and sharing of information between members of the multi-professional healthcare team*
- *helping to identify risks, and enabling early detection of complications*
- *supporting clinical audit, research, allocation of resources and performance planning, and*
- *helping to address complaints or legal processes.*

The principles of good record keeping set out by the NMC are shown in *Box 19.2* and would be relevant to all healthcare practitioners, not just nurses, midwives and health visitors.

Guidance is also provided in the former NHS Training Directorate booklets (NHS Training Directorate, 1995; HSC, 1998, 1999) and by the NHS Executive. The Audit Commission made recommendations to improve the standard of record keeping in hospitals in 1995 (Audit Commission, 1995). It reviewed the situation in 1999 and concluded that although progress had been made there was still scope for further improvements (Audit Commission, 1999).

The Clinical Negligence Scheme for Trusts, under the aegis of the NHS Litigation Authority, inspects the record keeping standards of those trusts who are members of the scheme and provides helpful guidance on standards.

Monitoring standards

Regular internal audit on record keeping standards is a useful method of identifying and maintaining standards. Internal audit can be supported by external reviews by the Kings Fund, other management consultancy organisations and the Care Quality Commission (see *Chapter 17*). To be effective the audit should be repeated at frequent intervals to identify if suggested changes are being implemented and standards improved.

Box 19.2 NMC Principles of good record keeping 2009

1. Handwriting should be legible.
2. All entries to records should be signed. In the case of written records, the person's name and job title should be printed alongside the first entry.
3. In line with local policy, you should put the date and time on all records. This should be in real time and chronological order and be as close to the actual time as possible.
4. Your records should be accurate and recorded in such a way that the meaning is clear.
5. Records should be factual and not include unnecessary abbreviations, jargon, meaningless phrases or irrelevant speculation.
6. You should use your professional judgement to decide what is relevant and what should be recorded.
7. You should record details of any assessments and reviews undertaken and provide clear evidence of the arrangements you have made for future and ongoing care. This should also include details of information given about care and treatment.
8. Records should identify any risks or problems that have arisen and show the action taken to deal with them.
9. You have a duty to communicate fully and effectively with your colleagues, ensuring that they have all the information they need about the people in your care.
10. You must not alter or destroy any records without being authorised to do so.
11. In the unlikely event that you need to alter your own or another healthcare professional's records, you must give your name and job title, and sign and date the original documentation. You should make sure that the alterations you make, and the original record, are clear and auditable.
12. Where appropriate, the person in your care, or their carer, should be involved in the record keeping process.
13. The language that you use should be easily understood by the people in your care.
14. Records should be readable when photocopied or scanned.
15. You should not use coded expressions of sarcasm or humorous abbreviations to describe the people in your care.
16. You should not falsify records.

Other principles are set out in relation to confidentiality, access, disclosure, information sytems and personal and professional knowledge and skills.

Prescribing

There are many decided cases where harm has been caused to a patient as a result of handwriting that has been misread by a pharmacist. For example, in one case (*Prendergast v Sam & Dee Ltd* [1989]) the doctor prescribed amoxil (an antibiotic) for the patient which, because of bad handwriting, was misread as daonil (a drug used by diabetics) by the pharmacist. As a consequence of the wrong medication the patient suffered from severe hypoglycaemia and brain damage from oxygen shortage in the blood. The doctor was held 25% to blame and the pharmacist 75%. The latter should have been alerted to the misreading because of the dosage and the fact that the patient paid for the prescription. £119 302 was paid out in compensation. In another case (Kennedy, 1996) a junior doctor and staff nurse misread the dose written up for a patient who had had a hysterectomy. The consultant had prescribed a top up epidural of 3 mg of diamorphine in 10 ml of saline; the junior doctor misread this as 30 mg. The patient died.

As more and more practitioners extend their professional roles to include prescribing powers, good handwriting will become essential. Eventually computer records and computer generated prescriptions may avoid the necessity for reliance on hand-written prescriptions and documentation.

A prescription

Advice is given in the *British National Formulary* on the writing of prescriptions.

> *Prescriptions*
> * *should be written legibly in ink or otherwise so as to be indelible,*
> * *should be dated,*
> * *should state the full name and address of the patient,*
> * *should be signed in ink by the prescriber.*
> *The age and the date of birth of the patient should preferably be stated and it is a legal requirement in the case of prescription-only medicine to state the age for children under 12 years.*

The *British National Formulary* also gives advice on the writing of dosages, the use of abbreviations and on computer-issued prescriptions. It notes that computer-generated facsimile signatures do not meet legal requirements.

Records used in pain management

Information about the pain suffered by the patient should be included in the following records:

- General observations of the patient's condition (often kept at the bedside).
- Nursing and medical records setting out treatment plans, prescription charts and pain scores and management.
- Audit records by pain practitioners often using pro formas or hand held computers.
- Specific records for patients on patient controlled analgesia (PCA).
- Specific records for epidural analgesia and patients with special problems.

The pain practitioner can have a valuable role in standard setting and monitoring by carrying out regular audit with ward colleagues on the completion of records and the recording of pain levels and pain management.

Application of the law to the situation in *Box 19.1*

It is apparent that the failure to record levels of pain suffered by the patient is a major defect in the record keeping standards of those caring for Marius. If there had been appropriate recording, it may have been that the failure to calibrate the syringe driver at the correct level would have come to light much earlier in the patient's treatment. The complaint would appear to be soundly based and the trust should ensure that an apology is given. It should also give an assurance that staff training will be undertaken to prevent such a mistake recurring.

Conclusions

Good standards of record keeping are part of the practitioner's professional duty of care to the patient. If a good standard is maintained in the clarity and comprehensiveness of the entries, then it is likely that, if there is a complaint, or litigation or other hearing, the documentation would provide adequate evidence for use before these hearings so as to explain the conduct and actions of the practitioner. However, like health and safety practice, there has to be constant monitoring to ensure that standards do not fall.

Questions and exercises

1. Examine the extent to which your and your colleagues' record keeping satisfies the standards of reasonable practice.
2. What differences would it make to your record keeping practice, if all patients were responsible for the safeguarding of their records?
3. How frequently is an audit carried out of record keeping standards in your department? Could it be made more effective?

References

Audit Commission (1995) *Setting the Records Straight: A Study of Hospital Medical Records*. Abingdon: Audit Commission

Audit Commission (1999) *Update Setting the Records Straight*. Abingdon: Audit Commission

HSC (1998) *Preservation, Retention and Destruction of GP Medical Services Records Relating to Patients*. 1998/217. London: HSC

HSC (1999) *For the Record: Managing Records in NHS Trusts and Health Authorities*. 1999/053. London: HSC

Kennedy D (1996) Hospital blamed in report on overdose death. *The Times* 3 July: 4

NHS Training Directorate (1995) *Just for the Record*. London: NHS Training Division

Nursing and Midwifery Council (2009) *Record Keeping: Guidance for Nurses and Midwives*. London: NMC

Prendergast v Sam & Dee Ltd [1989] 1 Med LR 36

CHAPTER 20

Research

Box 20.1 Situation

Ortis was employed as a pharmacist in a district general hospital. She was aware that a drug trial was taking place in the hospital on a new analgesic. She was dispensing this to a patient and asked the patient if she was aware that the drug was part of a research project. The patient stated that she had no knowledge of any such research but was taking the medicine for her arthritis. What should Ortis do?

Introduction

Research into both medications and treatment regimes is likely to become more and more a feature of patient care. Reasonable standards of care require that where possible research-based clinically effective practice is followed, which necessitates increasing random control testing for many procedures whose efficacy is assumed rather than established through clear research. As a consequence many pain practitioners might find that they themselves are involved in a research project, or if not, they are caring for patients who are the research subjects in a colleague's research project.

All the principles of law that have been considered in this book apply to the patient who is asked to participate in a research project. Of particular concern is the law relating to consent, confidentiality and liability if harm to the patient should occur, and this will be considered briefly here. The reader is referred to the list of further reading on p. 177 for detailed discussion on these and other legal issues. As part of the clinical governance initiative, the Department of Health published a research governance framework with the second edition published in May 2004 (Department of Health, 2001a, 2004). The framework sets out the responsibilities of a research sponsor and requires that organisations willing to take on these duties should be included on a list of recognised sponsors and complete a baseline assessment. The framework seeks to establish standards for all those involved in research in health and social care. In 2006 the Department of Health initiated a new programme for research in the NHS called *Best Research for Best Health*. The strategy and its implementation plans prepared by the new National Institute of Health Research (NIHR) can be downloaded from the Department of Health website (www.dh.gov.uk/).

Law relating to research

The Human Rights Act 1998 (see *Chapter 2*) and all other statutes and common law decisions also apply to the rights of data subjects. In addition there are statutory regulations for the carrying out of research on animals – Animals (Scientific Procedures) Act 1986, and for the testing of medicinal products – Medicines Act 1968, and for testing on embryos – Human Fertilisation and Embryology Act 1990.

Declarations and guidance

Many declarations from international conventions and guidelines from professional registration bodies or associations also cover research practice. However these declarations and guidelines, whilst they are frequently incorporated into the standards of professional practice, are not in themselves directly enforceable in the courts in this country. For example, two of the principle conventions covering the practice of research are the Nuremberg Code and the Declaration of Helsinki. Ten principles, which should be observed in order to satisfy moral, ethical and legal concepts, were laid down by the Nuremberg Courts following the military trials that took place at the end of the Second World War. These principles have become known as the Nuremberg Code (Kennedy and Grubb, 2000) and are summarised in *Box 20.2*.

Subsequently the World Medical Association published a Declaration of Helsinki in 1964 which set out principles for the carrying out of research on human subjects. Amendments were made in 2000 following a conference in Edinburgh (European Forum for Good Clinical Practice, 1999). Whilst the Declaration of Helsinki is not directly binding on the courts of this country (as the European Convention on Human Rights is through the Human Rights Act 1998), local ethics committees and researchers would have regard to its principles when giving agreement to and embarking on a research project.

Most health professional registration bodies and professional associations have drawn up guidelines for undertaking research. For example the Standards Committee of the General Medical Council (GMC) has drafted guidance entitled *Medical Research: The Role and Responsibilities of Doctors*, which is obtainable from the GMC website (www.gmc-uk.org/).

Consent

All those principles relating to the consent of the patient and the giving of information to the patient prior to any project starting (which are considered in *Chapters 6-10*) apply. Special provisions relate to any research on children and unless there are clear therapeutic benefits to a child, it is doubtful if a parent has the right in law to give consent on behalf of their children to research which

> ### Box 20.2 Principles for research from Nuremberg Code
>
> 1. The voluntary consent of the human subject is absolutely essential.
> 2. The experiment should be such as to yield fruitful results for the good of society, unprocurable by other methods.
> 3. The experiment should be based on results of animal experiments and a knowledge of the natural history of the disease or other problem so that the anticipated results should justify the performance of the experiment.
> 4. The experiment should be so conducted as to avoid all unnecessary physical and mental suffering and injury.
> 5. No experiment should be conducted where there is an a priori reason to believe that death or disabling injury will occur; except, perhaps, in those circumstances where the experimental physicians also serve as subjects.
> 6. The degree of risk to be taken should never exceed that determined by the humanitarian importance of the problem to be solved by the experiment.
> 7. Proper preparations should be made and adequate facilities provided to protect the experimental subject against even remote possibilities of injury, disability or death.
> 8. The experiment should be conducted only by a scientifically qualified person. The highest degree of skill and care should be required through all stages of the experiment of those who conduct or engage in the experiment.
> 9. During the course of the experiment the human subject should be at liberty to bring the experiment to an end if he has reached the physical or mental state where continuation of the experiment seems to him to be impossible.
> 10. During the course of the experiment the scientist in charge must be prepared to terminate the experiment at any stage, if he has probable cause to believe, in the exercise of the good faith, superior skill and careful judgment required of him, that a continuation of the experiment is likely to result in injury, disability, or death to the experimental subject.

may carry risks where these are not offset by therapeutic benefits. The United Nations Convention on the Rights of the Child was drawn up in 1989 and ratified by the UK in 1991. It represents clear guidance for the development of rights-based and child-centred healthcare.

There are advantages in a researcher obtaining the services of an independent person to explain the project and obtain a valid consent.

Research and those lacking capacity to give valid consent

As a consequence of the Mental Capacity Act (MCA) 2005 there are now statutory provisions covering research on those over 16 years who lack the capacity to give consent to research. The provisions do not cover research involving clinical trials, since those lacking capacity to consent are covered by the clinical trial regulations (Medicines for Human Use [Clinical Trials] Regulations 2004), enacted in 2004.

The MCA prohibits intrusive research being carried out on, or in relation to, a person who lacks the capacity to consent unless certain conditions are met. These conditions are shown in *Box 20.3*. Intrusive research is defined in section 30(2) as 'research which would be unlawful if carried out on a person capable of giving consent, but without that consent'.

The conditions laid down in Section 31 are shown in *Box 20.4*.

Box 20.3 Conditions required for research on those lacking the requisite mental capacity to give consent

- that the research is part of a research project,
- which is approved by an appropriate body as defined in Section 31,
- complies with the conditions laid down in Section 31 (see *Box 20.4*), and
- complies with conditions relating to the consulting of carers and additional safeguards (i.e. Sections 32 and 33 see below).

Box 20.4 Conditions for approval of a research project relating to a person lacking the capacity to consent (Section 31)

(2)   The research is connected with an impairing condition affecting P (the person lacking mental capacity) or its treatment.

(3)   An impairing condition is defined in Section 31(3) as a condition which is (or may be) attributable to, or which causes or contributes to, the impairment of, or disturbance in the functioning of, the mind or brain.

(4)   There must be reasonable grounds for believing that the research would not be as effective if carried out only on, or only in relation to, a person who has the capacity to consent to taking part in the project.

(5)(a) The research must have the potential to benefit P without imposing on P a burden that is disproportionate to the potential benefit to P or

(5)(b) be intended to provide knowledge of the causes or treatment of, or of the care of persons affected by, the same or a similar condition.

(6)   If (5)(b) applies and not (5)(a), there must be reasonable grounds for believing (a) that the risk to P from taking part in the project is likely to be negligible, and (b) that anything done to, or in relation to, P will not

    (i) interfere with P's freedom of action or privacy in a significant way, or

    (ii) be unduly invasive or restrictive.

(7)   There must be reasonable arrangements in place for ensuring that the requirements of Sections 32 and 33 are in place. (Consulting of carers and additional safeguards – see below).

Consulting of carers

The researcher 'R' is required to take reasonable steps to identify a person who is not engaged in a professional capacity nor receiving remuneration but is engaged in caring for P or is interested in P's welfare and is prepared to be consulted by the researcher under Section 32.

Subsection (7) makes it clear that the fact that a person is the donee of a lasting power of attorney given by P, or is P's deputy, does not prevent him or her from being the person consulted under Section 32.

If such a person cannot be identified, then R must, in accordance with guidance issued by the Secretary of State or the Welsh Assembly, nominate a person who is prepared to be consulted by R but has no connection with the project.

R must provide the carer or nominee with information about the project and ask him for advice as to whether P should take part in the project and what, in his opinion, P's wishes and feelings about taking part in the project would be likely to be if P had capacity in relation to the matter. If the person consulted advises R that in his opinion P's wishes and feelings would be likely to lead him to decline to take part in the project (or to wish to withdraw from it) if he had the capacity, then R must ensure that P does not take part, or if he is already taking part, ensure that he is withdrawn from taking part.

If treatment has commenced it is not necessary to discontinue the treatment if R has reasonable grounds for believing that there would be a significant risk to P's health if it were discontinued.

There are provisions under Section 32 Subsections 8 and 9 where treatment is to be provided as a matter of urgency and R considers that it is also necessary to take action for the purposes of the research as a matter of urgency, but it is not reasonably practicable to consult under the above provisions of this section. Under Subsection 9, the researcher, R, may take the action if

(a) he has the agreement of a registered medical practitioner who is not involved in the organisation or conduct of the research project, or

(b) where it is not reasonably practicable in the time available to obtain that agreement, he acts in accordance with a procedure approved by the appropriate body at the time when the research project was approved under Section 31.

However, the researcher may not continue to act in reliance on Subsection 9 if he has reasonable grounds for believing that it is no longer necessary to take the action as a matter of urgency.

There are additional safeguards to protect the interests of the person lacking the requisite mental capacity:

Nothing may be done to, or in relation to, a person taking part in the research project who is incapable of giving consent,

- *to which he appears to object (whether by showing signs of resistance or otherwise) except where what is being done is intended to protect him from harm or to reduce or prevent pain or discomfort, or*
- *which would be contrary to an advance decision of his which has effect or any other form of statement made by him and not subsequently withdrawn and R is aware of this.*

The MCA expressly states in Section 33(3) that the interests of the person must be assumed to outweigh those of science and society.

Special provisions apply if P had consented to take part in a research project begun before the commencement of Section 30 (1 April 2007) but, before the conclusion of the project, P loses capacity to consent to continue to take part in it. In such a situation regulations provide that despite his loss of capacity, research of a prescribed kind may be carried out on, or in relation to, P if:

- the project satisfies the prescribed requirements,
- any information or material relating to which is used in the research is of a prescribed description and was obtained before P's loss of capacity, and
- the person conducting the project takes such steps as may be prescribed for the purpose of protecting him.

Regulations (Mental Capacity Act 2005 [Loss of Capacity during Research Project] [England] Regulations 2007) covering the situation where an adult who had given consent to participation in research lost the requisite mental capacity during the research project were enacted in 2007. Further information on the Mental Capacity Act 2005 and its relevance to research and those lacking mental capacity can be found in Dimond (2007) and in the Code of Practice (Department of Constitutional Affairs, 2007).

Confidentiality

Information obtained from the patient during the research project is subject to exactly the same laws on confidentiality as those in *Chapter 12*. The same exceptions to the duty apply and justification for disclosure in the public interest would exist if serious harm to the patient or to other persons were feared.

Liability for harm

Even though the Pearson Report (Pearson, 1978) recommended that both volunteers and patients who take part in medical research and clinical trials and who suffer severe damage as a result should receive compensation on the basis of strict liability, this recommendation has never been implemented in law. Most research initiated by pharmaceutical companies is however conducted on the basis that compensation would be paid to those who were harmed as a result of participation in a research project and the local research ethics committee would ensure that this agreement was signed.

Local research ethics committees (LREC)

The Department of Health in 1991 requested each health authority ensures that an LREC was set up to examine research proposals. All those involved in research projects, whether as actual researchers or as carers for patients who are research subjects, were required to ensure that there has been LREC approval to the project. Some research is conducted on a multi-centred basis and multi-centre research ethics committees (MRECs), established by the Department of Health, oversee research which is carried on across several LREC catchment areas. Where less than five LRECs are involved, one LREC can act on behalf of the others. New arrangements for the appointment and work of the LRECs were published in 2001 and came into force in 2002 (Department of Health, 2001b). Further information on LRECs and the Government's research governance framework can be found on the Department of Health website (www.dh.gov.uk/).

Application of the law to the situation in *Box 20.1*

It is clear that there are real concerns to Ortis as to whether the patient has been given sufficient information about the medicines she is taking and the fact that she is participating in a research project. Ortis should raise these concerns with the doctor. It may well be that the research is being carried out on a multi-centre basis. However that is no justification for failing to ensure that each patient has been given the relevant information about the project and has given a valid consent. With support from her manager, Ortis could make it clear that the pharmacy department will not dispense medications that are being used on a trial basis, unless the patients have clearly been told about the research and have had an opportunity to consent to or refuse participation in the research.

Conclusions

There is a considerable range of guidance both international, national and professional on undertaking research. It may be that in future more of this guidance will be brought into legislation (as it is in respect of those lacking the requisite mental capacity to give consent) and become legally binding upon researchers and therefore more easily enforceable by the patient. The new patient organisations considered in *Chapter 18* are also likely to become involved in ensuring that research projects recognise and protect the rights of the patient. The openness and integrity called for by the Kennedy Report (2001) into paediatric heart surgery at Bristol should be at the heart of any research project.

Questions and exercises

1. How do you ensure that your practice keeps pace with accepted research findings?
2. If you were caring for a patient who was taking part in a research project what action would you take to ensure that the rights of the patient were protected?
3. You have been asked to assist in a research project. What issues would you clarify before you commenced your work?

References

Department for Constitutional Affairs (2007) *Code of Practice*. Available from: www.justice.gov.uk

Department of Health (1991) *Local Research Ethics Committees* HSG(91)5 1991

Department of Health (2001a) *Research Governance Framework*. Available from: www.doh.gov.uk/research/rd3/nhsrandd/researchgovernance.htm

Department of Health (2001b) *Governance Arrangements for NHS Research Ethics Committees*; replaces HSG(91)5 (the red book) and HSG(97)23 on multi-centre Research Ethics Committees. London: Department of Health

Department of Health (2004) *Research Governance Framework for England*, (2nd edn). Available from: www.doh.gov.uk/research/rd3/nhsandd/research-governance.htm

Department of Health (2006) *Best Research for Best Health*. London: Department of Health

Dimond B (2007) *Legal Aspects of Mental Capacity*. Oxford: Blackwell

European Forum for Good Clinical Practice (1999) *Bulletin of Medical Ethics Revising the Declaration of Helsinki: A fresh start*. London 3-4 September 1999

Kennedy I, Grubb A (2000) *Medical Law* (3rd edn) London: Butterworths

Kennedy Report (2001) *Bristol Royal Infirmary. Learning from Bristol: The report of the public inquiry into children's heart surgery at the Bristol Royal Infirmary 1984-1995* Command Paper CM 5207 July 2001. Available from: http://www.bristol-inquiry.org.uk/

Medicines for Human Use (Clinical Trials) Regulations 2004 SI 2004 No 1031

Pearson Lord (1978) *Royal Commission on Civil Liability and Compensation for Personal Injury Chaired by Lord Pearson.* Cmnd 7054 1978 HMSO

United Nations Convention on the Rights of the Child (1989) 20. Xi.1989; TS 44; Cm 1976

CHAPTER 21

Social security and other financial provisions

> **Box 21.1 Situation**
>
> Jim knows that he is likely to die very soon and wants to ensure that his relatives are not financially burdened by his care during his final weeks. He therefore wishes to find out the benefits to which he is entitled to ensure an application is made for these as soon as possible.

Introduction

There is a bewildering array of benefits available from Health Authorities, (for example, travelling expenses to hospital), from the Benefits Agency, the Department for Work and Pensions (in which there is a business unit known as the Disability and Carers Directorate), the Local Authority and the Department for Business, Innovation and Skills (which replaced the Department for Business Enterprise and Regulatory Reform, of which the Department of Trade and Industry was the predecessor). Each benefit has its own conditions of entitlement, some are backdated, some only payable from the date a claim has been made. Any person who gives advice in this area must ensure that it is up to date. It is preferable to give individuals the source of where advice can be obtained rather than pretend to have full comprehensive up-to-date knowledge. The internet is an invaluable source of advice and an A to Z guide to social security benefits is provided on the Social Security Agency's website (www.dsdni.gov.uk/index/ssa/benefit_information/a-z_of_benefits/).

The following information is only a brief outline of the benefits currently available and further details should be obtained from the relevant departments.

Benefits fall into one of four categories

1. Benefits available as of right.
2. Benefits available on a means tested basis either through social security or the local authority.

3. Benefits which are work related and eligibility depends upon meeting certain criteria relating to length of continuous service and other conditions laid down in the legislation.
4. Benefits available from a trust fund or charity

Benefits available to all

Disability Living Allowance (DLA)

This is part of the Disability and Carers Service and is available on a non-means tested basis for persons who are under 65 years and who need help with personal care or getting around because they are ill or disabled. It is paid at one of three levels. There is provision under Special Rules which enables a person to receive highest rate care without delay and without enduring a qualifying benefit. This is payable to a person who has a terminal illness and is not expected to live for more than 6 months. A mobility payment may also be made if a person is under 65 years and is applying for DLA under the Special Rules.

Attendance Allowance (AA)

This is available tax free for disabled people aged 65 and over who need help with personal care because of their illness or disability. Normally the help must have been needed for at least six months. Two rates of benefit are payable: a lower rate for day or night care or a higher rate for day and night care. The special provision (see above under DLA) for those with a terminal illness is also available under the Attendance Allowance.

Constant Attendance Allowance may be payable to someone who is receiving Industrial Injuries Disablement Benefit at the 95% rate or more because they need daily care and attendance. Constant Attendance Allowance is a tax-free benefit which is payable at one of four rates depending on the care needs. If Constant Attendance Allowance is paid at one of the two higher rates and the need for care is likely to be permanent the claimant may qualify for Exceptionally Severe Disablement Allowance.

Employment and Support Allowance

Incapacity benefit was available to those who are ineligible for the statutory sick pay scheme. From 27 October 2008 Employment and Support Allowance applied to new customers and replaced Incapacity Benefit and Income Support (paid on incapacity grounds). Existing customers will initially continue to receive their existing benefits so long as they continue to satisfy the entitlement conditions

Means tested benefits

Income Support

This was available to people on a low income, who are over 16 years and not working (or working less than 16 hours a week) but has been abolished by the Welfare Act 2009.

Working Families Tax Credit

Payable through the Inland Revenue as a deduction for tax payable in respect of working people who are bringing up children.

The Social Fund

Help is available with exceptional expenses which are hard to pay for out of regular income. A Community Care Grant, Budgeting Loan or Crisis Loan are available for specific purposes. The loans have to be paid back but are interest free. Funeral payments, cold weather payments and winter fuel payments are also payable to those on low incomes. A funeral payment is intended to help pay for certain funeral costs for those on a low income if they are responsible for arranging the funeral. It is recoverable from any money available from the deceased's estate.

Invalidity Care Allowance

This is available for persons between 16 and 65 who are spending at least 35 hours a week caring for a severely disabled person who is in receipt of the middle or highest level of DLA care component or AA.

Council tax benefit

Local authorities will reduce the amount payable in council tax by those who are on low incomes or who live on their own. Disabled people and carers may also receive discounts on council tax.

Housing Benefit

This is paid by the local council for people who need help with rent. The amount payable depends upon the means of the claimant, and the general level of rents in the area for that type of property.

Health Benefits

The following are available to specified groups or those on low incomes receiving income support:

- Free prescriptions
- Free NHS dental treatment
- Free NHS sight test
- Voucher towards cost of glasses or contact lenses
- Free NHS wigs and fabric supports
- Travel costs to and from hospital.

Work-related benefits

In addition there are benefits such as maternity payments and leave and statutory sick pay which are available for employees.

Benefits available from a trust fund or charity

The Charity Finance Yearbook, available in any public library, gives details of charitable organisations and trust funds that may be able to assist individuals who are in need.

Independent Living Fund

The Independent Living Fund is a trust set up to provide cash payments to severely disabled people. It offers severely disabled people the opportunity of living independently at home instead of in residential care by helping to pay towards the costs of their personal and/or domestic care. For full details contact the Independent Living Fund (PO Box 7525, Nottingham, NG2 4ZT; Funds@ ilf.org.uk; Tel: 0845 6018815).

Collection of benefits

Arrangements can be made for another person to collect benefit by nominating an appointee to be recognised by the local post office. Alternatively an official power of attorney can be submitted or the claimant can name another person whom they would like to receive their benefit on their behalf.

Application of the law to the situation in *Box 21.1*

Urgent advice should be obtained for Jim on the benefits that are available to him. If he is under 65 he may be able to eligible for Disability Living

Allowance and the special provision for those who are terminally ill. If he is over 65 then Attendance Allowance may be available as well as the allowance for the terminally ill.

Conclusions

Pain practitioners will find it useful to know who can be contacted to provide detailed advice to their patients. It may be that there is a social worker who specialises in benefits or a person within the benefit agency may be recommended to provide up-to-date expertise on the way through the benefits maze. At a time when a patient is gravely ill and facing death, it is essential that he or she does not have to cope with financial worries and uncertainties, and knowledgeable, speedy assistance is vital to the patient and his or her family. If contact is made with the local Department of Social Security office, it will endeavour to speed up any decision on benefits payable in the light of Jim's condition.

Questions and exercises

1. Find out where you can obtain up-to-date advice on benefits for patients receiving palliative care.
2. How can the interests of the patient be protected when relatives are obtaining the benefits on the patient's behalf? (You may need to seek the advice of the Benefits Agency on this.)
3. What are the legal consequences if you give misleading advice to patients which results in their losing some benefits to which they would have been entitled had they applied in time? (Refer also to *Chapters 4 and 10*)

CHAPTER 22

Conclusions

The second edition of this succinct book does not pretend to cover in detail all aspects of the law relating to pain management. The intention has been to introduce the law to those who are not familiar with its jargon and content and to provide a ready reference to others who need to refresh their knowledge.

It is hoped that practitioners will be able to follow up this book by referring to some of the more detailed works contained in the list of further reading on p. 177. Inevitably, new statutes are passed (for example, the Mental Capacity Act 2005 discussed in this second edition), new cases decided and the law moves on. It is therefore imperative, as in other aspects of their professional practice, that practitioners keep up to date with these changes. In addition practitioners are required to keep up with the guidance provided by their regulatory bodies and NHS organisations such as the Care Quality Commission, the National Service Frameworks, the National Patient Safety Agency and the National Institute for Health and Clinical Excellence. The findings from Inquiries might also be relevant to their practice. For example, a report chaired by Robert Frances QC which looked at failings in Mid-Staffordshire to provide basic patient care has made significant recommendations which are relevant to all practitioners (Department of Health, 2010). Palliative care practitioners will also find useful the reports of the National Confidential Enquiry into Patient Outcome and Death which are available on its website (www.ncepod.org.uk) and in particular its 2009 report, *Deaths in Acute Hospitals: Caring to the End?*

If this book has opened up a subject which is seen by many as forbidding and threatening and if it has enabled practitioners to pursue their work of pain management with greater confidence in using the law to protect their patients, their colleagues and themselves, then it will have served its purpose.

Reference

Department of Health (2010) *Independent Inquiry Into Mid Staffordshire NHS Foundation Trust*. London: Department of Health

National Confidential Enquiry into Patient Outcome and Death (2009) *Deaths in Acute Hospitals: Caring to the End?* Available from: www.ncepod.org. uk

Index of cases

A

B

C

D

F

G

H

J

K

M

P

R

S

W

X

Y

Index of statutes

P

S

W

Abbreviations

AA	Attendance Allowance
CHAI	Commission of Healthcare Audit and Inspection
CMP	Clinical Management Plan
CNHC	Complementary and Natural Healthcare Council
CPPIH	Commission for Patient and Public Involvement in Health
CPS	Crown Prosecution Service
CPSM	Council for the Professions Supplementary to Medicine
CQC	Care Quality Commission
DLA	Disability Living Allowance
DPP	Director of Public Prosecutions
GMC	General Medical Council
HASWA	Health and Safety at Work Act 1974
HPC	Health Professions Council
HSC	Health and Safety Commission
HSE	Health and Safety Executive
IMCA	Independent Mental Capacity Advocate
LINK	Local Involvement Network
LREC	Local Research Ethics Committee
MCA	Medicines Control Agency
MDA	Medical Devices Agency
MHRA	Medicines and Healthcare Products Regulatory Agency
MREC	Multi-Centre Research Ethics Committee
MRI	Magnetic Resonance Imaging
NCI	NHS Centre for Involvement
NICE	National Institute for Health and Clinical Excellence
NIHR	National Institute of Health Research
NMC	Nursing and Midwifery Council
NPSA	National Patient Safety Agency
NSF	National Service Frameworks
PALS	Patient Advocacy and Liaison Service
PCA	Patient Controlled Analgesia
RIDDOR	Reporting of Injuries, Diseases and Dangerous Occurrences (Regulations) 1995
SHA	Strategic Health Authority
UKCC	United Kingdon Central Council for Nursing, Midwifery and Health Visiting

Glossary

A

accusatorial a system of court proceedings where the two sides contest the issues (*contrast with* **inquisitorial**)

Act of Parliament, **statute**

actionable per se a court action where the claimant does not have to show loss, damage or harm to obtain compensation, e.g. an action for **trespass to the person**

actus reus the essential element of a crime which must be proved to secure a conviction, as opposed to the mental state of the accused (***mens rea***)

adversarial the approach adopted in an **accusatorial** system

advocate a person who pleads for another: it could be paid and professional, such as a **barrister** or **solicitor**, or it could be a lay advocate either paid or unpaid

assault a threat of unlawful contact (trespass to the person)

B

balance of probabilities the standard of proof in civil proceedings

barrister a lawyer qualified to take a case in court

battery an unlawful touching (*see* **trespass to the person**)

best interests anything done for people without capacity must be in their best interests (there is no legal definition of best interests, but the criteria to be used are in Section 4 of the Mental Capacity Act 2005). Best interests means that thinking about what is best for the person, not about what anyone else wants

Bolam Test the test laid down by Judge McNair in the case of *Bolam v. Friern HMC* on the standard of care expected of a professional in cases of alleged negligence

burden of proof the duty of a party to litigation to establish the facts, or in criminal proceedings the duty of the prosecution to establish both the *actus reus* and the *mens rea*

C

case law judge-made law

cause of action the facts that entitle a person to sue

civil action proceedings brought in the civil court

civil wrong an act or omission which can be pursued in the civil courts by the person who has suffered the wrong (*see* **tort**)

committal proceeding hearings before the magistrates to decide if a person should be sent for trial in the crown court

common law law derived from the decisions of judges

conditional fee system a system whereby client and lawyer can agree that payment of fees is dependent upon the outcome of the court action

coroner a person appointed to hold an inquiry (inquest) into a death in unexpected or unusual circumstances

criminal wrong an act or omission which can be pursued in the criminal courts

D

damages a sum of money awarded by a court as compensation for a **tort** or breach of contract

declaration a ruling by the court, setting out the legal situation

dissenting judgment a judge who disagrees with the decision of the majority of judges

distinguished (of cases) the rules of precedent require judges to follow decisions of judges in previous cases where these are binding upon them. However in some circumstances it is possible to come to a different decision because the facts of the earlier case are not comparable to the case now being heard, and therefore the earlier decision can be 'distinguished'

E

ex gratia as a matter of favour, e.g. without admission of liability, of payment offered to a claimant

expert witness evidence given by a person whose general opinion based on training or experience is relevant to some of the issues in dispute

H

hierarchy the recognised status of courts which results in lower courts following the decisions of higher courts (*see* **precedent**). Thus decisions of the House of Lords must be followed by all lower courts unless, they can be distinguished (see above)

I

indictment a written accusation against a person, charging him or her with a serious crime, triable by jury

injunction an order of the court restraining a person

inquisitorial a system of justice whereby the truth is revealed by an inquiry into the facts conducted by the judge, e.g. **coroner**'s court

J

judicial review an application to the High Court for a judicial or administrative decision to be reviewed and an appropriate order made, e.g. declaration

L

litigation civil proceedings

M

magistrate a person (Justice of the Peace or stipendiary magistrate) who hears summary (minor) offences or indictable offences which can be heard in the magistrates court

mens rea the mental element in a crime (*contrast with* **actus reus**)

O

obiter dicta (literally latin – remarks in passing) something said by a judge while giving judgment that was not essential to the decision in the case. Contrasts with *ratio decidendi*

ombudsman a Commissioner (e.g. health, Local Government) appointed by the Government to hear complaints

P

plaintiff term formerly used to describe one who brings an action in the civil courts. Now the term claimant is used

practice direction guidance issued by the head of the court to which they relate on the procedure to be followed

precedent a decision which may have to be followed in a subsequent court hearing (see **hierarchy**)

prima facie at first sight, or sufficient evidence brought by one party to require the other party to provide a defence

privilege in relation to evidence, being able to refuse to disclose it to the court

proof evidence which secures the establishment of a claimant's or prosecution's or defendant's case

prosecution the pursuing of criminal offences in court

Q

quantum the amount of compensation, or the monetary value of a claim

R

ratio decidendi (literally latin – the reason for deciding) the principles of law on which the court relies in deciding a case. To be distinguished from *obiter dicta*

Re F ruling a professional who acts in the best interests of an incompetent person who is incapable of giving consent, does not act unlawfully if he or she follows the accepted standard of care according to the **Bolam Test**

reasonable doubt to secure a conviction in criminal proceedings the prosecution must establish beyond reasonable doubt the guilt of the accused

S

solicitor a lawyer who is qualified on the register held by the Law Society

statute law (statutory) law made by **Acts** of Parliament

strict liability liability for a criminal act where the mental element does not have to be proved; in civil proceedings liability without establishing negligence

subpoena an order of the court requiring a person to appear as a witness (*subpoena ad testificandum*) or to bring records/documents (*subpoena duces tecum*)

summary offence a lesser offence which can only be heard by a **magistrate**

T

tort a civil wrong excluding breach of contract. It includes: negligence, **trespass** (to the person, goods or land), nuisance, breach of statutory duty and defamation

trespass to the person a wrongful direct interference with another person. Harm does not have to be proved

U

ultra vires outside the powers given by law (e.g. of a statutory body or company)

vicarious liability the liability of an employer for the wrongful acts of an employee committed whilst in the course of employment

Appendix I

Schedule 1 to the Human Rights Act 1998

Articles of the European Convention on Human Rights

Part I

The Convention
Rights and Freedom

Article 2
Right to life

1. Everyone's right to life shall be protected by law. No one shall be deprived of his life intentionally save in the execution of a sentence of a court following his conviction of a crime for which this penalty is provided by law.
2. Deprivation of life shall not be regarded as inflicted in contravention of this Article when it results from the use of force which is no more than absolutely necessary:
   (a) in defence of any person from unlawful violence;
   (b) in order to effect a lawful arrest or to prevent the escape of a person lawfully detained;
   (c) in action lawfully taken for the purpose of quelling a riot or insurrection.

Article 3
Prohibition of torture

No one shall be subjected to torture or to inhuman or degrading treatment or punishment.

Article 4
Prohibition of slavery and forced labour

1. No one shall be held in slavery or servitude.
2. No one shall be required to perform forced or compulsory labour.
3. For the purpose of this Article the term 'forced or compulsory labour' shall not include:
   (a) any work required to be done in the ordinary course of detention imposed according to the provisions of Article 5 of this Convention or during conditional release from such detention;
   (b) any service of a military character or, in case of conscientious objectors in countries where they are recognised, service exacted instead of

compulsory military service;
  (c) any service exacted in case of an emergency or calamity threatening the life or well-being of the community;
  (d) any work or service which forms part of normal civic obligations.

Article 5
Right to liberty and security

1. Everyone has the right to liberty and security of person. No one shall be deprived of his liberty save in the following cases and in accordance with a procedure prescribed by law:
  (a) the lawful detention of a person after conviction by a competent court;
  (b) the lawful arrest or detention of a person for non-compliance with the lawful order of a court or in order to secure the fulfilment of any obligation prescribed by law;
  (c) the lawful arrest or detention of a person effected for the purpose of bringing him before the competent legal authority on reasonable suspicion of having committed an offence or when it is reasonably considered necessary to prevent his committing an offence or fleeing after having done so;
  (d) the detention of a minor by lawful order for the purpose of educational supervision or his lawful detention for the purpose of bringing him before the competent legal authority;
  (e) the lawful detention of persons for the prevention of the spreading of infectious diseases, of persons of unsound mind, alcoholics or drug addicts or vagrants;
  (f) the lawful arrest or detention of a person to prevent his effecting an unauthorised entry into the country or of a person against whom action is being taken with a view to deportation or extradition.
2. Everyone who is arrested shall be informed promptly, in a language which he understands, of the reasons for his arrest and of any charge against him.
3. Everyone arrested or detained in accordance with the provisions of paragraph 1(c) of this Article shall be brought promptly before a judge or other officer authorised by law to exercise judicial power and shall be entitled to trial within a reasonable time or to release pending trial. Release may be conditioned by guarantees to appear for trial.
4. Everyone who is deprived of his liberty by arrest or detention shall be entitled to take proceedings by which the lawfulness of his detention shall be decided speedily by a court and his release ordered if the detention is not lawful.
5. Everyone who has been the victim of arrest or detention in contravention of the provisions of this Article shall have an enforceable right to compensation.

Article 6
Right to a fair trial

1. In the determination of his civil rights and obligations or of any criminal charge against him, everyone is entitled to a fair and public hearing within a reasonable time by an independent and impartial tribunal established by law. Judgment shall be pronounced publicly but the press and public may be excluded from all or part of the trial in the interest of morals, public order or national security in a democratic society, where the interests of juveniles or the protection of the private life of the parties so require, or to the extent strictly necessary in the opinion of the court in special circumstances where publicity would prejudice the interests of justice.

2. Everyone charged with a criminal offence shall be presumed innocent until proved guilty according to law.

3. Everyone charged with a criminal offence has the following minimum rights:
    (a) to be informed promptly, in a language which he understands and in detail, of the nature and cause of the accusation against him;
    (b) to have adequate time and facilities for the preparation of his defence;
    (c) to defend himself in person or through legal assistance of his own choosing or, if he has not sufficient means to pay for legal assistance, to be given it free when the interests of justice so require;
    (d) to examine or have examined witnesses against him and to obtain the attendance and examination of witnesses on his behalf under the same conditions as witnesses against him;
    (e) to have the free assistance of an interpreter if he cannot understand or speak the language used in court.

Article 7
No punishment without law

1. No one shall be held guilty of any criminal offence on account of any act or omission which did not constitute a criminal offence under national or international law at the time when it was committed. Nor shall a heavier penalty be imposed than the one that was applicable at the time the criminal offence was committed.

2. This Article shall not prejudice the trial and punishment of any person for any act or omission which, at the time when it was committed, was criminal according to the general principles of law recognised by civilised nations.

Article 8
Right to respect for private and family life

1. Everyone has the right to respect for his private and family life, his home and his correspondence.

2. There shall be no interference by a public authority with the exercise of this right except such as is in accordance with the law and is necessary in a democratic society in the interests of national security, public safety or the economic wellbeing of the country, for the prevention of disorder or crime, for the protection of health or morals, or for the protection of the rights and freedoms of others.

Article 9
Freedom of thought, conscience and religion
1. Everyone has the right to freedom of thought, conscience and religion; this right includes freedom to change his religion or belief and freedom, either alone or in community with others and in public or private, to manifest his religion or belief, in worship, teaching, practice and observance.
2. Freedom to manifest one's religion or beliefs shall be subject only to such limitations as are prescribed by law and are necessary in a democratic society in the interests of public safety, for the protection of public order, health or morals, or for the protection of the rights and freedoms of others.

Article 10
Freedom of expression
1. Everyone has the right to freedom of expression. This right shall include freedom to hold opinions and to receive and impart information and ideas without interference by public authority and regardless of frontiers. This Article shall not prevent States from requiring the licensing of broadcasting, television or cinema enterprises.
2. The exercise of these freedoms, since it carries with it duties and responsibilities, may be subject to such formalities, conditions, restrictions or penalties as are prescribed by law and are necessary in a democratic society, in the interests of national security, territorial integrity or public safety, for the prevention of disorder or crime, for the protection of health or morals, for the protection of the reputation or rights of others, for preventing the disclosure of information received in confidence, or for maintaining the authority and impartiality of the judiciary.

Article 11
Freedom of assembly and association
1. Everyone has the right to freedom of peaceful assembly and to freedom of association with others, including the right to form and to join trade unions for the protection of his interests.
2. No restrictions shall be placed on the exercise of these rights other than such as are prescribed by law and are necessary in a democratic society in the interests of national security or public safety, for the prevention of disorder or crime, for the protection of health or morals or for the protection of the

rights and freedoms of others. This Article shall not prevent the imposition of lawful restrictions on the exercise of these rights by members of the armed forces, of the police or of the administration of the State.

Article 12
Right to marry

Men and women of marriageable age have the right to marry and to found a family, according to the national laws governing the exercise of this right.

Article 14
Prohibition of discrimination

The enjoyment of the rights and freedoms set forth in this Convention shall be secured without discrimination on any ground such as sex, race, colour, language, religion, political or other opinion, national or social origin, association with a national minority, property, birth or other status.

Article 16
Restrictions on political activity of aliens

Nothing in Articles 10, 11 and 14 shall be regarded as preventing the High Contracting Parties from imposing restrictions on the political activity of aliens.

Article 17
Prohibition of abuse of rights

Nothing in this Convention may be interpreted as implying for any State, group or person any right to engage in any activity or perform any act aimed at the destruction of any of the rights and freedoms set forth herein or at their limitation to a greater extent than is provided for in the Convention.

Article 18
Limitation on use of restrictions on rights

The restrictions permitted under this Convention to the said rights and freedoms shall not be applied for any purpose other than those for which they have been prescribed.

Part II

The First Protocol

Article 1
Protection of property

Every natural or legal person is entitled to the peaceful enjoyment of his possessions. No one shall be deprived of his possessions except in the public interest and subject to the conditions provided for by law and by the general principles of international law.

The preceding provisions shall not, however, in any way impair the right of a State to enforce such laws as it deems necessary to control the use of property in accordance with the general interest or to secure the payment of taxes or other contributions or penalties.

Article 2
Right to education

No person shall be denied the right to education. In the exercise of any functions which it assumes in relation to education and to teaching, the State shall respect the right of parents to ensure such education and teaching in conformity with their own religious and philosophical convictions.

Article 3
Right to free elections

The High Contracting Parties undertake to hold free elections at reasonable intervals by secret ballot, under conditions which will ensure the free expression of the opinion of the people in the choice of the legislature.

Part III

The Sixth Protocol

Article 1
Abolition of the death penalty

The death penalty shall be abolished. No one shall be condemned to such penalty or executed.

Article 2
Death penalty in time of war

A State may make provision in its law for the death penalty in respect of acts committed in time of war or of imminent threat of war; such penalty shall be applied only in the instances laid down in the law and in accordance with its provisions. The State shall communicate to the Secretary General of the Council of Europe the relevant provisions of that law.

Websites

Action for Advocacy	www.actionforadvocacy.org
Action on Elder Abuse	www.elderabuse.org.uk
Advisory Conciliation and Arbitration Service	www.acas.org.uk
Age Concern	www.ageconcern.org.uk
Alert	www.donoharm.org.uk
Alzheimer's Research	www. Alzheimers-research.org.uk
Alzheimer's Society	www.alzheimers.org.uk
ASA Advice	www.advice.org.uk
Association of Contentious Trust and Probate Solicitors	www.actaps.com
Audit Commission	www.audit-commission.gov.uk
Bailii (case law resource)	www.bailii.org/ew/cases
Bristol Royal Infirmary Inquiry	www.bristol-inquiry.org.uk/
Care Quality Commission	www.cqc.org.uk
Care Services Improvement Partnership	www.csip.org.uk
CARERS UK	www.carersonline.org.uk
	www.carersuk.org
Central Office for Research Ethics Committees	www.corec.org.uk
Citizen Advocacy Information and Training	www.citizenadvocacy.rg.uk
Citizens Advice Bureaux	www.citizensadvice.org.uk
Civil Procedure Rules	www.open.gov.uk/lcd/civil/procrules_fin/crules.htm
Clinical Negligence Scheme for Trusts	www.nhsla.com/Claims/Schemes/CNST/
Commission for Patient and Public Involvement in Health	www.cppih.org/
Commission for Racial Equality	www.cre.gov.uk/
Commission for Social Care and Inspection	www.csci.gov.uk
Community Legal Service Direct	www.clsdirect.org.uk
Complementary and Natural Healthcare Council	www.cnhc.org.uk

Complementary Healthcare Information Service	www.chisuk.org.uk
Contact the Elderly	www.contact-the-elderly.org
Convention on the International Protection of Adults	www.hcch.net/index_en.php?
Council for Healthcare Regulatory Excellence	www.chre.org.uk
Counsel and Care	www.counselandcare.org.uk
Court Funds Office	www.hmcourts-service.gov.uk/ infoabout/cfo/index.htm
Court of Protection	via the Office of Public Guardian or HM Courts Services
Dementia Care Trust	www.dct.org.uk
Department for Business Enterprise and Regulatory Reform	www.berr.gov.uk/employment
Department for Education and Skills	www.dfes.gov.uk
Department for Work and Pensions	www.dwp.gov.uk/
Department of Health	www.dh.gov.uk
Department of Trade and Industry	www.dti.gov.uk/
Disability Law Service	www.dls.org.uk/
Domestic Violence	www.domesticviolence.gov.uk
Down's Syndrome Association	www.downs-syndrome.org.uk www.dsa-uk.com
Equality and Human Rights Commission	www.equalityhumanrights.com
Family Carer Support Service	www.familycarers.org.uk
Family Mediation Helpline	www.familymediationhelpline.co.uk
Foundation for People with Learning Disabilities	www.learningdisabilities.org.uk
General Medical Council	www.gmc-uk.org
Headway – Brain Injury Association	www.headway.org.uk
Health and Safety Commission	www.hsc.gov.uk
Health and Safety Executive	www.hse.gov.uk
Healthcare Commission	www.healthcarecommission.org.uk/
Health Professions Council	www.hc-uk.org

Help the Aged	www.helptheagedorg.uk
Help the Hospices	www.hospiceinformation.info
HM Courts Service	www.hmcourts-service.gov.uk
Home Farm Trust	www.hft.org.uk
Human Fertilisation and Embryology Authority	www.hfea.gov.uk/
Human Genetics Commission	www.hgc.gov.uk
Human Rights	www.humanrights.gov.uk
Independent Mental Capacity Advocate	www.dh.gov.uk.imca
Independent Safeguarding Authority	www.isa-gov.org.uk
Information Commissioner's Office	www.ico.gov.uk
Law Centres Federation	www.lawcentres.org.uk
Law Society	www.lawsociety.org.uk/ choosingandusing/findingasolicitor.law
Legal cases (England and Wales)	www.bailli.org/ew/cases
Legislation	www.opsi.gov.uk/legislation or www.legislation.hmso.gov.uk
Linacre Centre for Healthcare Ethics	www.linacre.org
Making Decisions Alliance	www.makingdecisions.org.uk
Manic Depression Fellowship	www.mdf.org.uk
MedicAlert Foundation	www.medicalert.org.uk
Medicines and Healthcare Products Regulatory Agency	www.mhra.gov.uk
MENCAP	www.mencap.org.uk
Mental Capacity Implementation Programme	www.dca.go.uk/legal-policy/mental-capacity/index.htm
Mental Health Act Commission	www.mhac.org.uk/
Mental Health Foundation	www.mentalhealth.org.uk
Mental Health Lawyers Association	www.mhla.co.uk
Mental Health Matters	www.mentalhealthmatters.com/
Mind	www.mind.org.uk
Ministry of Justice	www.justice.gov.uk
Motor Neurone Disease Association	www.mndassociation.org.uk
National Audit Office	www.nao.gov.uk

National Autistic Society   www.nas.org.uk
                                                  www.autism.org.uk
National Care Association   www.nca.gb.com
National Confidential Enquiry into
      Patient Outcome and Death   www.ncepod.org.uk
National Family Carer Network   www.familycarers.org.uk
National Health Service Litigation
      Authority   www.nhsla.com
National Information and Governance
      Board for Health and Social Care   www.nigb.nhs.uk
National Mediation Helpline   www.nationalmediationhelpline.com
National Patient Safety Agency   www.npsa.gov.uk
National Perinatal Epidemiology Unit www.npeu.ox.ac.uk/
National Treatment Agency   www.nta.nhs.uk/
NHS   www.nhs.uk
NHS Direct   www.nhsdirect.nhs.uk
NHS Institute for
      Innovation and Improvement   www.institute.nhs.uk/
NHS Professionals   www.nhsprofessionals.nhs.uk
NICE   www.nice.org.uk
Nursing and Midwifery Council   www.nmc-uk.org/

Office of Public Guardian   www.guardianship.gov.uk
Office of Public Sector Information   www.opsi.gov.uk
Official Solicitor   www.officialsolicitor.gov.uk
Open Government   www.open.gov.uk

Pain   www.pain-talk.co.uk
Patient Concern   www.patientconcern.org.uk
Patient's Association   www.patients-association.org.uk
People First   www.peoplefirst.org.uk
Prevention of Professional
      Abuse Network   www.popan.org.uk
Princess Royal Trust for Carers   www.carers.org/

Relatives and Residents Association   www.releres.org/
RESCARE (The National Society
      for mentally disabled people
      in residential care)   www.rescare.org.uk
Respond   www.respond.org.uk
Rethink (formerly the National
      Schizophrenia Fellowship)   www.rethink.org
Royal College of Nursing   www.rcn.org.uk

Royal College of Psychiatrists	www.rcpsych.ac.uk
SANE	www.sane.org.uk
Scope	www.scope.org.uk
Sense	www.sense.org.uk
Solicitors for the Elderly	www.solicitorsfortheelderly.com
Speaking Up	www.speakingup.org/
Speakability	www.speakability.org.uk
Shipman Inquiry	www.the-shipman-inquiry.org.uk/reports.asp
Social Security Agency's A to Z guide to social security benefits	www.dsdni.gov.uk/index/ssa/benefit_information/a-z_of_benefits/
Stroke Association	www.stroke.org.uk
Together: Working for Wellbeing	www.together-uk.org
Turning Point	www.turning-point.co.uk
UK Homecare Association	www.ukhca.co.uk
UK Parliament	www.parliament.uk
United Response	www.unitedresponse.org.uk
Values into Action	www.viauk.org
Veterans Agency	www.veteransagency.org.uk
VOICE UK	www.voiceuk.clara.net
Voluntary Euthanasia Society	www.ves.org.uk
Welsh Assembly Government	www.wales.gov.uk
World Medical Association	www.wma.net/e/policy/b3.htm

Further reading

Appelbe GE, Wingfield J (eds) (2001) *Dale and Appelbe's Pharmacy: Law and Ethics* (7th edn) London: The Pharmaceutical Press

Beauchamp TL, Childres JF (2001) *Principles of Biomedical Ethics* (5th edn) Oxford: Oxford University Press

Benn P (1998 reprinted 2005) *Ethics*. Oxford: Routledge

Blom-Cooper L, Grounds A, Guinan P, Parker A, Taylor M (1996) *The Case of Jason Mitchell: Report of the Independent Panel of Inquiry*. London: Duckworth

Blom-Cooper L, Hally H, Murphy E (1996) *The Falling Shadow – One patient's mental health care 1978–1993* (Report of an Inquiry into the death of an occupational therapist at Edith Morgan Unit, Torbay 1993). London: Duckworth

Brazier M (2007) *Medicine, Patients and the Law* (4th edn) London: Penguin

Brazier M, Murphy J (eds) (2003) *Street on Torts*. (12th edn) London: Butterworth

British Medical Association (1998) *Medical Ethics Today*. London: BMJ Publishing

Campbell AV (1984) *Moral Dilemmas in Medicine*. Edinburgh: Churchill Livingstone

Card R (1998) *Cross and Jones' Criminal Law* (14th edn) London: Butterworth

Carey P (2004) *Data Protection: A practical guide to UK and EU law* (2nd edn) Oxford: Oxford University Press

Carson D, Bain A (2008) *Professional Risk and Working with People: Decision making in health, social care and criminal justice*. London: Jessica Kingsley Publishers

Clements L (2000) *Community Care and the Law* (2nd edn) London: Legal Action Group

Committee of Experts Advisory Group on AIDS (1994) *Guidance for Health Care Worker's Protection Against Infection with HIV and Hepatitis*. London: HMSO

Cooper J, Vernon S (1996) *Disability and the Law*. London: Jessica Kingsley Publishers

Cooper J (ed) *Occupational Therapy and Mental Health* (3rd edn) Edinburgh: Churchill Livingstone

Denis IH (1999) *The Law of Evidence*. London: Sweet and Maxwell

Department of Health (1993) *AIDS/HIV Infected Health Care Workers*. London: Department of Health

Dimond BC (1996) *Legal Aspects of Child Health Care*. London: Mosby

Dimond BC (1997) *Legal Aspects of Care in the Community*. London: Macmillan

Dimond BC (1997) *Mental Health (Patients in the Community) Act 1995: An introductory text*. London: Mark Allen

Dimond BC (1998) *Legal Aspects of Complementary Therapy Practice*. Edinburgh: Churchill Livingstone

Dimond BC (1999) *Patients' Rights, Responsibilities and the Nurse* (2nd edn) Central Health Studies. London: Quay Books

Dimond BC (2002) *Legal Aspects of Patient Confidentiality*. London: Quay Books

Dimond BC (2002) *Legal Aspects of Patient Confidentiality*. London: Quay Books

Dimond BC (2002) *Legal Aspects of Pain Management*. London: Quay Books

Dimond BC (2004) *Legal Aspects of Heath and Safety*. London: Quay Books

Dimond BC (2005) *Legal Aspects of Medicines*. London: Quay Books

Dimond BC (2005) *Legal Aspects of Midwifery* (3rd edn) London: Books for Midwives Press/Butterworth Heinemann

Dimond BC (2007) *Legal Aspects of Death*. London: Quay Books

Dimond BC (2007) *Legal Aspects of Mental Capacity*. Oxford: Blackwells Publishing

Dimond BC (2008) *Legal Aspects of Nursing* (5th edn) London: Pearson

Dimond BC (2009) *Legal Aspects of Consent* (2nd edn) London: Quay Books

Dimond BC (2009) *Legal Aspects of Physiotherapy* (2nd edn) Blackwell Science

Dimond BC (2010) *Legal Aspects of Occupational Therapy* (3rd edn) in press

Dimond BC, Barker F (1996) *Mental Health Law for Nurses*. Oxford: Blackwell Science

Doyle BJ (1996) *Disability Discrimination: The New Law*. Bristol: Jordans

Ellis N (1994) *Employing Staff* (5th edn) London: British Medical Association

Faulder C (1985) *Whose Body Is It?* London: Virago

Finch J (ed) (1994) *Speller's Law Relating to Hospitals* (7th edn) London: Chapman and Hall Medical

Fletcher N, Holt J (1995) *Ethics, Law and Nursing*. Manchester:Manchester University Press

Gann R (1993) *The NHS A to Z* (2nd edn) Winchester: The Help for Health Trust

Gibson C, Grice J, James R, Mulholland S (2001) *The Children Act Explained*. London: The Stationery Office

Glover J (1984) *Causing Death and Saving Lives*. London: Penguin

Glover J (1984) *What Sort of People Should There Be?* London: Penguin

Grainger I, Fealy M, Spencer M (2000) *Civil Procedure Rules in Action* (2nd edn) London: Cavendish Publishers

Ham C (1991) *The New National Health Service*. London: National Association of Health Authorities & Trusts

Harris P (2007) *An Introduction to Law* (7th edn) London: Butterworths

Health and Safety Commission (1999) *Management of Health and Safety at Work Regulations Approved Code of Practice*. London: HMSO.

Health and Safety Commission (1992) *Manual Handling Regulations and Approved Code of Practice*. London: HMSO

Health and Safety Commission (1992) *Guidelines on Manual Handling in the Health Services*. London: HMSO

Hendrick J (2006) *Law and Ethics in Nursing and Healthcare* (2nd edn) Cheltenham: Nelson Thornes Publishers

Herring J (2006) *Medical Law and Ethics*. Oxford: Oxford University Press

Heywood F (2001) *Money Well Spent: The effectiveness and value of housing adaptations*. Bristol: The Policy Press for Joseph Rowntree Foundation.

Hoggett B (2005) *Mental Health Law* (5th edn) London: Sweet and Maxwell

Howells G, Weatherill S (1995) *Consumer Protection Law*. Aldershot: Dartmouth Publishing

Hunt G, Wainright P (eds) (1994) *Expanding the Role of the Nurse*. Oxford: Blackwell Publishing

Hurwitz B (1998) *Clinical Guidelines and the Law*. Oxford: Radcliffe Medical Press

Ingman T (1996) *The English Legal Process* (6th edn) London: Blackstone Publishing

Jay R, Hamilton A (1999) *Data Protection Law and Practice*. London: Sweet and Maxwell

Jones MA (2007) *Textbook on Torts* (9th edn) Oxford: Oxford University Press

Jones R. (2009) *Mental Health Act Manual* (12th edn) London: Sweet and Maxwell

Keenan D (2007) *Smith and Keenan's English Law* (13th edn) Harlow: Longman

Kennedy T (1998) *Learning European Law*. London: Sweet and Maxwell

Kennedy I, Grubb A (2000) *Medical Law* (3rd edn) London: Butterworth

Kidner R (1993) *Blackstone's Statutes on Employment Law* (3rd edn) London: Blackstone Press

Kloss D (2000) *Occupational Health Law* (3rd edn) Oxford: Blackwell Publishing

Knight B (1992) *Legal Aspects of Medical Practice* (5th edn) Edinburgh: Churchill Livingstone

Leathard A, McLaren S (eds) (2007) *Ethics: Contemporary challenges in health and social care*. Bristol: The Policy Press

Lee RG, Morgan D (2001) *Human Fertilisation and Embryology Act 1990*. London: Blackstone Press

Leigh-Pollit P, Mullock J (2001) *The Data Protection Act Explained* (3rd edn) London: The Stationery Office

Mandelstam M (1997) *Equipment for Older or Disabled People and the Law*. London: Jessica Kingsley

Mandelstam M (1998) *An A-Z of Community Care Law*. London: Jessica Kingsley Publishers

Mandelstam M (2009) *Community Care Practice and the Law* (4th edn) London: Jessica Kingsley

Mason D, Edwards P (1993) *Litigation: A Risk Management Guide for Midwives*. London: Royal College of Midwives

Mason JK, McCall-Smith A (2010) *Law and Medical Ethics* (8th edn) London: Butterworths

McHale J, Fox M (2007) *Health Care Law* (2nd edn) London: Sweet and Maxwell

McHale J, Tingle J (2007) *Law and Nursing* (2nd edn) London: Elsevier Health Sciences

Metzer A, Weinberg J (1998) *Criminal Litigation*. London: Legal Action Group

Miers D, Page A (1990) *Legislation* (2nd edn) London: Sweet and Maxwell

Miles A, Hampton J, Hurwitz B (2000) *NICE, CHI and the NHS Reforms – Enabling excellence or imposing control?* London: Aesculapius

Montgomery J (2003) *Health Care Law* (2nd edn) Oxford: Oxford University Press

Murphy J (2006) *Street on Torts* (12th edn) London: Butterworths

National Association of Theatre Nurses (1993) *The Role of the Nurse as First Assistant in the Operating Department*. Harrogate: NATN

Oliver P (2003) *The Student's Guide to Research Ethics*. Maidenhead: Open University Press

Pearse P, et al (1988) *Personal Data Protection in Health and Social Services* London: Croom Helm

Pitt G (2000) *Employment Law* (4th edn) London: Sweet and Maxwell

Pyne RH (1991) *Professional Discipline in Nursing Midwifery and Health Visiting* (2nd edn) Oxford: Blackwell Publishing

Richards P (2009) *Law on Contract*. (9th edn) London: Financial Times and Pitman Publishing

Royal College of Nursing (1992) *Focus on Restraint* (2nd edn) London: RCN

Rowson R (1990) *An Introduction to Ethics for Nurses*. London: Scutari Press

Rowson R (2006) *Working Ethics – How to be fair in a culturally complex world*. London: Jessica Kingsley

Rumbold G (1993) *Ethics in Nursing Practice* (2nd edn) London: Baillière Tindall

Salvage J. (1988) *Nurses at Risk: Guide to Health and Safety at Work*. Heinemann London.

Salvage J, Rogers R (1988) *Health and Safety and the Nurse*. London: Heinemann

Saunders P (1989) *The A-Z of Disability Directory of Information Services Organisations Equipment and Manufacturers*. Marlborough: The Crowood Press Ramsay

Seedhouse D (2003) *Ethics: The Heart of Health Care*. Chichester: Wiley

Sellars C (2002) *Risk Assessment with People with Learning Disabilities*. Oxford: Blackwell Publishing

Selwyn N (1982) *Selwyn's Law of Safety at Work*. London: Butterworth

Selwyn N (2000) *Selwyn's Law of Employment* (11th edn) London: Butterworth

Sims S (2000) *Practical Approach to Civil Procedure* (4th edn) London: Blackstone Press

Skegg PDG (1998) *Law, Ethics and Medicine* (2nd edn) Oxford: Oxford University Press

Slapper G, Kelly D (2006) *The English Legal System* (8th edn) London: Routledge-Cavendish Publishing

Smith K, Keenan D (1992) *English Law* (10th edn) London: Pitman

Social Security Inspectorate Department of Health (1993) *No Longer Afraid: Safeguard of Older People in Domestic Settings*. London: HMSO

Stauch M, Wheat K, Tingle J (2002) *Source Book on Medical Law* (2nd edn) London: Cavendish Publishing

Steiner J (1992) *Textbook on EC Law* (3rd edn) London: Blackstone Press

Stone R (2009) *The Modern Law of Contract* (6th edn) London: Cavendish

Stone J, Matthews J (1996) *Complementary Medicine and the Law*. Oxford: Oxford University Press

Taylor MC (2000) *Evidence-Based Practice for Occupational Therapists*. Oxford: Blackwell Publishing

Tingle J, Cribb A (eds) (1995) *Nursing Law and Ethics* (3rd edn) Oxford: Blackwell Publishing

Tolley (2003) *Tolley's Health and Safety at Work Handbook* (15th edn) Croydon: Tolley

Tschudin V (2002) *Ethics in Nursing: The caring relationship* (3rd edn) London: Butterworth-Heinemann

Vincent C et al (1993) *Medical Accidents*. Oxford: Oxford University Press

Vincent C (ed) (1995) *Clinical Risk Management*. London: BMJ

Warnock M (2002) *An Intelligent Person's Guide to Ethics*. London: Duckworths

Watt H (2000) *Life and Death in Healthcare Ethics – A short introduction*. London: Routledge

Wheeler J (2002) *The English Legal System*. Harlow: Pearson Education

White R, Carr P, Lowe N (2002) *A Guide to the Children Act 1989* (3rd edn) London: Butterworth

Wilkinson R, Caulfield H (2000) *The Human Rights Act: A Practical Guide for Nurses*. London: Whurr Publishers

Young AP (1989) *Legal Problems in Nursing Practice*. London: Harper & Row

Young AP (1994) *Law and Professional Conduct in Nursing* (2nd edn) London: Scutari Press

Zander M (1995) *Police and Criminal Evidence Act* (3rd edn) London: Sweet and Maxwell

Index